HOMEOPATHIC
COLOR
REMEDIES

Other books by Ambika Wauters:

Healing with The Energy of The Chakras,
  The Crossing Press, Freedom, California, 1998.

Chakras and Their Archetypes,
  The Crossing Press, Freedom, California, 1997.

The Chakra Oracle,
  Conari Press, Berkeley, California, 1996.

The Angel Oracle,
  St. Martin's Press, New York, 1995.

The Principles of Color Healing,
  Harper-Collins, London, 1997.

HOMEOPATHIC COLOR REMEDIES

By Ambika Wauters, R. S. Hom.

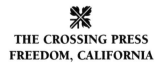

THE CROSSING PRESS
FREEDOM, CALIFORNIA

For information on bulk purchases or group discounts for this and
other Crossing Press titles, please contact our Special Sales
Manager at 800-777-1048.

Visit our Website on the Internet at: www.crossingpress.com

Library of Congress Cataloging-in-Publication Data
Wauters, Ambika.
   Homeopathic color remedies / by Ambika Wauters.
     p. cm.
   ISBN 0-89594-997-0
   1. Color--Therapeutic use. 2. Chakras. 3. Healing--Miscellanea.
4. Homeopathy--Materia medica and therapeutics I. Title.
   RZ414.6.W38 1999
   615.8'9--dc21   98-55114
                                          CIP

Acknowledgments

My gratitude to my teachers at the School of Homeopathic Medicine, Ian Townsend, Azziza Griffin, Bob Fordham, and Gill Scott, for their excellent teaching and for their high levels of personal integrity. My love to Jude Creswell, R. S. Hom., for her friendship and belief in me as a homeopath during years of study. She helped to soothe the struggle and doubt that are built into any training. To my agent, Susan Mears, who felt that a broader reading audience would benefit from this book and took it forward. Gratitude to Elaine Gill, founder of The Crossing Press, who saw the creative flame in me, gave it recognition, and space to flourish. What a gracious gift!

Table of Contents

Preface

Ambika asked me to write this preface because I have been rather closely involved with the development of these remedies almost from the beginning.

Color has been known for millennia to have a strong influence on people, and treatment with colored light has been used in naturopathic circles for several decades. One very funny story I heard in this connection was about a patient who was feeling very agitated and tense and the final advice her herbalist-naturopath gave her was to surround herself with blue. The next appointment was held at the patient's house, and the practitioner was astonished to find the whole house had been redecorated, so that paintwork, wallpaper, and soft furnishings were all blue! She had forgotten that the patient was enormously rich and could easily manage such redecoration—she had only meant that she should *imagine* herself surrounded with blue. But the blue had the desired effect, and the lady relaxed.

What is new in this book is to turn colors into potentized remedies, for use by homeopaths and others who give remedies in potency. This idea has required a big leap of acceptance even by homeopaths, but why should this be so?

As Ambika argues so well in her introductory chapter, all matter is energy, of waveforms from the longest to the shortest. If remedies can be made from minerals, plants, and animal sources, from solids, liquids, and gases and even from x-rays and other radioactive elements, then why not from colors, which occupy a part of the total wave spectrum?

Such was her premise, and this book is the first record of her researches into the effects of the various colors of the visible spectrum once potentized.

In homeopathy, information is gathered on the effect of possible remedies by testing them on healthy human volunteers. Many of us have tried out various colors in this way. Frankly, I did not believe that I would experience anything, but that night I had a dream in which the entire scene was tinted, even people's clothes, in the color that I was unknowingly proving at the time! So my skepticism was unfounded, and I was convinced by the strongest of testimonials, namely personal experience.

Others are now engaged in a series of very thorough homeopathic provings of these remedies, so that over an extended period of time and through a very careful collation of all the provers' notes of their experiences, a very detailed symptom picture will become available of all the colors. Then it is to be hoped that these remedies will find their way into general acceptance, as they will be able to be prescribed according to well-documented symptom pictures.

Meanwhile, we have what for many of us has been the long-awaited opportunity to study this book and get a comprehensive overview of the color remedies. As practitioners and healers we need to be open-minded and receptive to whatever discoveries may help us to be more effective in our art, which is trying to restore the sick to health.

This book is proof that Ambika Wauters is innovative and full of insight. She is not content just to follow in the steps marked out by others, nor is she limited just to the processes of rational thought. She does not get her knowledge out of books, but, directly from people. She is presenting to us in this book not only collated information about the colors and their effects but also her acquired wisdom concerning the makeup of humankind.

It is a privilege for me to have been asked to write this short preface, but even more now to be able to turn the pages and try to perceive and understand what is being offered to us here in this book.

Roger Savage
Saffron Walden, U.K.

Introduction

What a joy to live and breathe. Through all life we experience light and embrace color without even knowing how powerful its effects are on the way we think, move, feel, and function. We have been given such a wealth of healing power in light and color. It makes life and the processes of living virtually possible at the most basic levels. Without light there would not be any life on our planet as we know it to be. Plants could not survive, nor could any animal species.

When we are deprived of light our entire organism contracts and we shrivel, both physically and emotionally. In parts of the planet where people are deprived of light for long periods of time their bodily functions are transformed, and their habits and behavior are distinctly different. Eskimos do not become pregnant during the long harsh winters; their bodies are incapable of sustaining life at freezing temperatures and in the near darkness they endure through the long winters. When the light returns to the arctic tundra, life emerges. Cycles are re-established and procreation happens. This is a function of light as well as temperature.

At an emotional level we speak about love in terms of what warms us. We acknowledge warmhearted people and colorful characters as important for our emotional and mental life. Our simple language is full of words which describe light and color in people, places, and events. We are emerged in the flavor of colors and the love of light without conscious awareness of our intimate relationship with it.

I have always loved color from the time I was a small child. I would choose special colors of crayons to draw with and gave colors emotional codes even then. I was so certain about colors that I knew which ones would work together to form beautiful patterns and to describe the visions I had in my head. Little did I realize that, when homeopathy called me as a way of offering a very real method of healing, color would come to play a significant role in my understanding of healing. I used to imagine there was a place where art and healing came together. I now feel, in the color remedies, we may have that marriage.

When I wrote *The Principles of Color Healing* I meant it to be an introduction to how color could make our lives richer and an explanation of how colors could affect us. I had been doing homeopathic provings (the word we use in homeopathy for experiment) for several years when I began to write the basic introduction, but didn't feel that this material could be included in the book.

The material in this book is designed to take the inquisitive and higher mind further in the exploration of how powerful light and color are in providing us with a source of healing. Here we view the dynamic effect of potentized energy and learn how the quintessential energetic pattern of substance can have a profound effect on how we think, feel, and function. This book presents the evidence that light in potency can transform our behavior, play havoc with our dreams, and definitely promote our body to perform its daily functions more economically. It suggests that we are not the mechanical creatures we have been led to believe, but rather creatures of light, responsive to vibrational healing using color and sound.

For those who are unfamiliar with homeopathy, it is the treatment of symptoms with highly diluted substances. It is based on the underlying principle that "like cures like." This means that if you have a symptom, which could be physical, mental, or emotional, you can treat that symptom with a remedy which, in its proving, creates symptoms similar to your own. Coffee is a good example. If I gave you a strong cup of black coffee to drink, you might develop an upset stomach, begin to sweat, have loose bowels, find yourself unable to sleep, or become irritable and aggressive. If you came to see me as a homeopath and these were your presenting symptoms, I might give you homeopathic coffee, highly diluted of course, for the treatment of those symptoms. This is an ancient and effective way of treating illness.

The founder of homeopathy was Samuel Hahnemann, who lived in Germany at the end of the 19th century. His unique contributions to healing were the treatment of illnesses using this principle ("like cures like") and the element of dynamic potentization.

This process is achieved by making a series of dilutions of a substance chosen to treat the symptoms. It is scientifically prescribed method followed universally by homeopaths. The principles which Hahnemann created for prescribing and treating chronic and acute illness have not changed for over 250 years and are wonderfully effective in the treatment of all diseases, conditions, and states of emotional and mental distress. There are no harmful side effects to this form of treatment, as there is no toxic substance left after the series of dilutions which create the remedy.

People respond well to this form of treatment because it is safe, gentle, and effective. It is prescribed individually so that two people who might suffer from the same condition might need to receive two different remedies. Each person has their own unique way of being out of balance. For example, you may have your headache on the right side of your head, while someone else, who is also complaining of a headache, would have symptoms on the left, or at the back of the neck. This is a simplification of homeopathy, but it is meant to describe to the lay person that it is a highly differentiated form of healing.

Uniting the love of color and homeopathy has been very interesting for me personally. I intuitively understood the principles of homeopathy from the beginning of my studies. I also understood color without realizing the powerful potential it had to actually change physical and emotional states of being. The proving of color as a homeopathic medicine has been illuminating. I have seen instant changes in people experiencing distress. Many of the people who took the remedies in the provings shared similar dreams and had similar emotional experiences. It was possible from the very first day to know that potentized color could provide healing at a very real level.

One day while visiting a homeopathic tutor, she complained of a headache and was going to take a remedy. I suggested she try a color remedy. She was given Violet 6x and within minutes the symptoms disappeared. She gave me a very strange look and asked, "What is this stuff?"

The principles seem so simple to me but, whenever I explained it to homeopaths or my tutors, they would dismiss it as perhaps too simple or too obtuse. I have lived and worked with these remedies for nine years now, and I have witnessed wonderful healing with them. When Jan Scholten suggested that I do additional provings and get this information out to the homeopathic community, I gathered my courage and got to work.

This small book represents ten years of study, provings, and development at a professional and personal level. When I first saw that these remedies had healing powers, I wanted to share my knowledge with everyone. Many established homeopaths dismissed the healing properties of color and thought my work was extreme and unconventional. Homeopathy makes many remedies out of poisons and earthly substances. Light and color fall into the category of what are known as the imponderables. Many homeopaths felt this was an area into which they did not want to probe. At the beginning no one wanted to listen to a first-year student who had a great deal to learn about the nature of homeopathy.

However, in the provings done over the last ten years, it became evident that this form of homeopathy and vibrational healing could work effectively with some very impressive physical, mental, and emotional results. This book is designed to provide an accurate description of how potentized light and color can be used. The provings are described and a list of therapeutics is also provided in this book.

These remedies can be purchased through the homeopathic pharmacies or from the author. Give this book careful study before you decide that these remedies are something you would like to use. Although we are working with light we need to be as respectful of its power as we would be of more toxic substances. When you realize how we are affected by color and light you will be more aware of its ability to heal and how, in a dynamic or potentized form—which is what homeopathy is—we can transform our health.

How the Colors Were Made

The original color remedies were made at the Winter Solstice of 1989 in the Lake District of northern England. They were the result of an offhanded inquiry made during a homeopathic tutorial with homeopath Ian Watson, when, as a first-year student of classical homeopathy, I asked him how remedies were made. He replied that remedies could be made out of any substance on our planet. I asked if they could be made out of color. He said theoretically that was possible. He suggested that I try making some and see if they worked.

I thought this was a wonderful way to understand the homeopathic process. At the time, I had only a great deal of enthusiasm and very little knowledge. Over the years the ratio inverted. I gained knowledge and lost a great deal of that original enthusiasm, which was the spark that set the whole process in motion. There were times, over the years, the light nearly went out altogether. At one point, I threw away the original proving material because no one I knew was interested in them. I could get no assistance or support and just let the project linger on the back burner of my mind while I continued my studies. The time and energy it took to do provings and collate the material by myself, with little funding, made it an unattractive task. I have learned that very creative projects can rest unattended for years, simmering and stewing while you work on other things. The project stayed there for what felt like long, fallow periods. Then something would happen that would show me the power of these remedies, or someone would want to know how they worked and would offer assistance with another proving. It wasn't until, at the end of 1996, when I met the Dutch homeopath, Jan Scholten, that I had the impetus to go further. He was warm and full of enthusiasm for homeopathy, and he had developed a new way of looking at minerals and the periodic table. Meeting him and studying his approach to homeopathy rekindled the spark. I was fortunate that there was good support for doing more provings amongst a few homeopaths I knew. So we "got on with it," as they say in Britain.

When Ian Watson gave me the original impetus to make the first batch of remedies, I was left thinking how to make them. I had a dream shortly after the tutorial in which I was shown how to physically make the remedies. I gathered all the equipment I needed; distilled water, theatrical lighting gels in full spectrum colors, small cosmetic mirrors which could be tied around the containers, and beakers. Since I couldn't find any pink filters, I used a pair of pink silk tights to wrap around the containers as a source of color.

I made the first batch of remedies on the Winter Solstice, December 21, 1989. This is the day of minimal light in the northern hemisphere. Where I lived, in the north of England, there are only five hours of available light at that time of year. That day, the sky was overcast and the weather so dreary that I had no idea if the color would be absorbed into the water, nor did I know if the remedies would have any healing effect.

The remedies were originally preserved in vodka, as pure spirits were impossible to obtain. I then wondered how I was going to find anyone to prove them when two friends from college, Dave Evans and Greg Cornforth, came to visit and asked if they could have a drop of color to test out. I gave them Pink and sent them home after tea and a chat. The next day Dave called to tell me he thought I should look into these remedies. He reported that two patches of eczema in the creases of his elbows, which had persisted for a long time, suddenly disappeared overnight and, coincidentally, he had a fight with his partner, which was unusual as they shared a normally tranquil relationship.

I suddenly began searching for people who would be willing to take the remedies and tell me what they experienced. This is how material is gathered in homeopathy. It is called a proving. The results of the first provings were extremely encouraging. I went to a Buddhist retreat center and asked for volunteers. I also asked students at the Fellside Alexander Technique School in Kendal, Cumbria, if they would act as provers. There were also some students or friends who were willing to take the risk and try the remedies. Hahnemann said, in his treatise on homeopathic provings, that the best people to use for provings were those people who lived and shared the same conditions, who followed the same daily routines; ate the same food, and drank the same water for long periods of time. I was fortunate that two such communities were available near me, and both communities were comprised of self-aware and open people who were willing to help me.

The original results really were amazing. A nun from the Buddhist center who had suffered from rheumatoid arthritis for forty years was relieved from pain as a result of taking one dose of Indigo 30x. She immediately developed boils along the liver meridian of both legs. When I asked another prover, who took the same color, if anything unusual had happened to him, he told me that six women had fallen in love with him that week. I asked if this was part of his normal experience, and to what did he attribute this experience. He said that he felt his confidence was extremely high while on the remedy. This same prover also dared to dive off nearby cliffs into the sea. This was something he feared more than anything and had been looking for courage to do for over a year. He felt, while on the remedy, that he could do anything he wanted.

This original proving of Indigo 30x led me to conclude that the pituitary gland was affected by the remedy. One prover, who was a sedentary, cold, woman in her fifties, suffered great emotional distress on the remedy. She felt acutely detached and disconnected and went to her general practitioner and asked to be given drugs to alleviate her misery.

This was the beginning of differentiating the remedies and finding prescribable symptoms. Blue has proven to increase the suffering of depressive people. The expression to "have the blues" seems to come from an deep unconscious knowledge about the character of this color. Blue gives clarity of mind and detachment to those embroiled in life. It also helps to lessen our engagement with people and situations. It proved to be healing for this woman because it forced her to ground her energies. She began having regular massage, as she longed for touch. It also forced her to reach out to others and ask for help, something she had never done before.

After this experience, however, I decided the best way to test these imponderable remedies was in clinical provings. In a clinical situation, people could have healing rather than be used as guinea pigs while I sought to discover how the remedies worked. In the beginning I decided to dowse for which color would best suit the patient. From there I was able to establish, from the complaints and types of emotional issues people faced, which remedies worked for what conditions.

I had reports from over twenty provers that a wide variety of symptoms occurred to them while taking the remedies. Some of the colors had very clear physical characteristics, while others seemed to work more subtly on emotional and mental levels. For instance, a very interesting thing happened to all the provers who took Pink. They all dreamed of being with their mothers, or of motherhood. These dreams were always soothing and comforting. One woman, who was pregnant and contemplating a termination, decided to go ahead with the pregnancy after taking the color. Pink was obviously about mother love.

As I began to be inundated with data I was able to see how these color remedies worked on different levels. They differed from conventional color healing, which used light and pigment, because they touched deeper into the energetic economy of the patient. The most obvious information about the colors was that they worked in relation to the chakras or energy centers of the body. These are non-anatomical energy points located in the subtle energy sheath we call the aura. They channel vital energy into the physical body and act as conductors, or filters, of energy which comes up from the earth and down from the cosmos. Where these two energies meet forms a vertex, known as a chakra. These two energies are part of the electromagnetic scale. The magnetic is earth energy and is red; the electric energy is from the cosmos and is blue.

The chakras correspond to colors, sounds, emotional issues, and archetypes, and are present in all organic life forms. I began to explore the nature of chakras in 1990 and, by 1993, had published the first of four books on the chakras, their emotional components, and life issues. These books explore the nature of these energy centers and how positive thought, energy massage, and awareness can transform our energy and strengthen our chakras.

The second and third books explore the archetypes of empowerment, vitality, and responsibility as they correspond to the chakras. Color relates to the chakras and plays an important part in rebalancing and realigning our energy. The chakras are a focal point for shifting energetic and emotional blocks, and color contributes to this transformation in a major way. Homeopathic color remedies act as a medicine for our energy body.

I received considerable help in doing the provings, and I would like to say a special thanks to Roger Savage, R.S. Hom., and Liz Kinsey, R.S. Hom., both colleagues of Scholten and longstanding homeopaths in Britain. Roger was very supportive throughout the ten years of provings and encouraged me when others were not forthcoming. He asked me to speak about my findings at the Society of Homoeopaths annual meeting in 1997 and, from there, other homeopaths expressed their interest and support. Cheryl Conran-Brown, R.S. Hom., and Maxine Fawcett, two homeopaths living near me, agreed to supervise provers. The provers came from friends, patients, and interested people to whom I am deeply grateful. My gratitude extends to all those willing people who took the initial batch of color remedies and who gave me the awareness that these were indeed powerful healing tools. Melissa Assilem, R. S. Hom., invited a clairvoyant friend to read the energy of the remedies many years ago, and we were all amazed that her blind awareness of the energy is completely consistent with the findings of many old, established color healers.

Provings are a time-consuming job and require a great deal of responsibility. The supervising homeopaths took the provers' cases and checked with them at least once a day for three weeks to gather new symptoms, check old symptoms, and assess the cases of the provers. This was done without money and with substantial goodwill on their part. I appreciate everything that they did to follow the protocol for provings.

Officially Potentizing the Colors

The remedies were officially potentized by John Morgan and his staff at Helios Pharmacy in Tunbridge Wells, Kent, England, in early 1992. We are now using the stock remedies they made. When the remedies were taken to Helios we had two batches: one made at the Winter Solstice, and another made at the Summer Solstice. We dowsed to see which batch had the strongest energy field. What we found was interesting. The hot colors of Red, Orange, and Yellow were strongest in the Winter Solstice batch. Green, Turquoise, Indigo, and Violet were the strongest from the Summer Solstice batch. Nature gave her warmth when it was coldest, and her coolness when it was hot. Magenta and Spectrum were the same in both batches. We took the strongest colors from batches and made our remedies from them.

They were potentized at Helios by Catherine Bolderstone, a homeopath who since that time has developed a deep interest in color. She kept an account of her personal process while making the remedies. Her personal journal, written during the time she made the remedies into various potencies, reads like a fairytale. While working on the process she met her husband, was courted, and married. Shortly thereafter she had her first baby.

The remedies are now seven years old and are ready to be used by both homeopaths and the lay public. They can be used knowing that they are gentle, safe, and effective in the treatment of physical, mental, and emotional symptoms. They are similar to the flower essences as they work to rebalance disharmonious energy states. They penetrate into the physical realm of pathology and can be given for physical complaints as well as for emotional healing or spiritual insight. It is my opinion that these remedies work best when used in conjunction with deep-acting homeopathic mineral remedies, such as homeopathic hormonal remedies and constitutional remedies. Hormones also address the chakras and are closely aligned to colors. I give colors to support the action of a constitutional remedy.

In their mode of action the potentized color remedies fit somewhere between the flower essences and homeopathic plant remedies; they are supportive and work in specific realms of mind/body/spirit. They can, however, work well on their own, particularly for spiritual insight and emotional harmony.

Clinical Provings

All the provings which have been done recently have been provings in clinical situations where the remedy was indicated for the patient and used to treat clinical symptoms. A classical homeopathic case was addressed, and the patient's emotional presentation of symptoms indicated which chakras were out of balance. Using the color of that chakra, I arrived at the appropriate color remedy.

Other ways to diagnose which color remedy is required is to look at the organs affected, and the area of the body where the symptoms are located. Understanding the emotional issues a person is currently addressing in their life will also lead you to the chakra and, hence, to the color required.

In the provings, each prover kept a notebook for three weeks in which they wrote how they felt spiritually, mentally, emotionally, and physically. The prover's observations were analyzed in depth by a homeopath. The remedy was then given in three split doses over 24 hours and each day the homeopath and the prover discussed everything the prover could remember happening throughout that 24-hour period. Based on the symptoms noted from three weeks of journal entry and the discussions between the prover and homeopath after the remedy was taken, the supervising homeopath would ascertain whether the symptoms were new or old ones.

In every case the color remedy helped the prover in some significant way. This was seen at physical, mental, and emotional levels. The results indicated to me that the ongoing process of psychological and spiritual development can be enhanced by the use of colors to stimulate a weak or overactive chakra.

I found it was more useful to give a color remedy that was indicated by clinical diagnosis for specific symptoms than to randomly prove a color in an experiential sense. I had unusual results when I gave a remedy without a clinical diagnosis. For example, one redheaded prover, in the early days of provings, took Red and tried to kill her husband with a dinner fork by stabbing him in the chest. Red was not the color this already inflamed woman needed. She would have experienced healing with the cooler colors, although we would never have known how powerful Red could be on the emotions had she not taken it. Another highly volatile prover threw all his wife's best china against a wall in a rage. He did not need the hot color of Orange but rather something more soothing to sedate his fiery temperament. I soon realized these hot people needed cooling down, not fueling up. This was a very pragmatic way in which I learned how color remedies worked.

The color remedies used in the recent provings were chosen by various methods. In some cases they were dowsed for, but in others the emotional issues the patient was facing indicated the color very clearly. At other times the patient felt drawn to a particular color which was revealed in taking the case history. The different ways of finding the right color are discussed in this book.

In my experience these remedies offer us a unique way of letting light provide us with the gift of healing. By potentizing light, we bring the quintessential vibration of energy into play with our bodies and spirits and let it work to rebalance and recharge us. Light and color are food for our nerves, blood, and tissue, as well as for our souls. They also feed our emotions and mental states, as we have witnessed throughout the provings.

The remedies can also provide us with a model for self-awareness, helping us to understand ourselves better. By understanding the colors and the chakra system, we can see our own psychological and developmental issues more clearly. This helps us take greater responsibility for who we are and where our energy is fixed or arrested. For instance, if we are having problems with confidence, the color indicated is Yellow because it relates to the Solar Plexus, the chakra which relates to our personal power and issues of confidence and self-worth. As a former psychotherapist and healer, I see that the qualities these remedies stimulate can provide balance and harmony. They can open doors to our awareness of who we are and help us honor our worth.

This book is modeled after Jan Scholten's book, *Homoeopathy and Minerals*. I felt this was a simple and easy way to understand new information. It will provide the reader with a succinct way of working with the content of this book. The format will illustrate how each color works in terms of its physical, emotional, mental, and spiritual properties. It also gives some background material which may be interesting for the reader.

I am grateful to the colors which fill my life with meaning and which have allowed me a channel of personal and professional expression. Without color, my world would be very dim, and the wonders and beauty of life would be lacking the enchantment they hold for me.

I wish the international homeopathic community pleasure and success in healing. I hope these color remedies add to the wonderful work you are doing. This is also extended to healers the world over who are finding the extraordinary benefits of color in their practice.

I would appreciate any feedback which can help us understand colors and their healing properties. Please write to me if you would like to share your experiences of these remedies. Likewise, you can order remedies from me should you wish. A few years ago the homeopathic pharmacy discarded all the color remedies by accident, and I am now making my own supplies. Please write, fax, or email the publisher and your request will be forwarded on to me.

May your life be rich and colorful, a full color spectrum of experiences.

The Nature of Color
and the Human Energy System

"The universe is filled with color."

—Sir Isaac Newton—

This quote appears at the entrance of the Jodrell Bank Telescope Laboratory. Color captured the imagination of Sir Isaac Newton, one of the great scientific minds in history.

We own our understanding of the fundamental properties of light to him. Color, however, has been used for healing since ancient times. It is known that the early Egyptians bounced light off of prisms to focus color onto parts of the body. It is said that they developed colors which cannot be created to this day. The ancients employed color to balance and heal the mind/body/spirit. They not only understood its physical properties but also respected the esoteric aspects of color. They put into practice their knowledge of color through the ministrations of priestesses and healers, who taught initiates how to develop their spiritual powers through the use of color. That we are again using color for healing reawakens our deepest potential for growth and self-development. We now have an advanced technology which allows us to break down color into energy, and we are also developing the wisdom to know how to use light as medicine in both allopathic and homeopathic form. There are now advances in the use of light and color in both fields of medicine. This book will open your eyes to the healing properties of homeopathic color remedies and give you insight into how you might find healing for yourself with their use.

Color and Life

Color is fundamental to life. Color vibrations are necessary for our physical growth and development. Color exists in the form of oscillating light waves which, when viewed through the energy spectrum, are broken down into the components of white light. When we look at the emanations of energy that come from cosmic rays as they enter the earth's atmosphere, we see that white light is only a small portion of a greater energy. The electromagnetic scale, which is how modern scientists measure the cosmic forces as they penetrate our earth's atmosphere, begins with gamma rays, which oscillate at a particular speed and vibrate at a fixed rate. As these vibrations slow down, they become X-rays, again with their own fixed patterns of movement and vibration. As this energy slows down even more, it becomes ultraviolet light. In the next step in the process of deceleration energy becomes visible white light, which further breaks down into the colors of the spectrum. As these waves of energy slow even more they become infrared waves, then microwave, radar, FM radio, television, short wave, and, finally, AM radio waves.

When we understand the full range of the electromagnetic spectrum we can begin to understand our own homeopathic materia medica better. All substances, or remedies, fit into this spectrum of light, energy, and color. Knowledge about this scale of energy helps us understand where each of the remedies fits into the scale of vibration.

We can also understand the color our patients need for their healing. Sometimes we see people who are "out of it." They hover in the realms of the cosmic forces and are not fully physical or incarnate. They lack the red energy of life and can appear as pale shades of blue or violet. We look for remedies which will ground these people and bring back their natural vitality; remedies which will put them back into the colorful flow of life. These are often the patients who do well on Camphor or Coca, which, in the spectrum of color, fit into the blue and violet part of the spectrum. We are following the principle of "like curing like" when we give them the remedy which carries those high and unearthed vibrations.

At other times we see people who are too earthed; too fired by the passions of life. They lack refinement, and their bodies are plagued with the diseases of lower vibrations, which fall into the red or orange part of the spectrum. You can imagine that their pathology tends towards inflammation, problems with disorganization of the blood and vital energy.

Sometimes we see people who would benefit from more earthy elements, such as the orange light, who need greater sexuality, or more appetite for life. At other times we need to assist people in finding their spiritual nature, which is a higher color or vibration. They need more of the violet or magenta and less of the earthy colors of red and orange.

All our homeopathic remedies have their place on this scale of energy and color. It is really a way of looking at color in relation to our patients' needs that can help facilitate their healing and balance. As we explore the nature of their symptoms, we can see into which band of color or energy they fit, and which colors will help them move forward in their life. How we see that color can be translated into a homeopathic remedy, a herbal tincture, or even a vitamin.

The electromagnetic scale contains the energy we need for balancing not only ourselves but all life forms on our planet. Where a person's energy fits on this scale can give us information about what needs healing in an individual and how we can best provide that healing. This is where vibrational medicine becomes a part of the universal energy force which can aid in adjusting and retuning our energy fields.

As we use these energetic forces for healing the vibrational field of people, so our planet will shift to a higher vibration of energetic resonance and will create greater harmony within the energetic economy of the planet itself.

It is interesting that most of the remedies we now use in homeopathy fall into the color range of yellow to lime green. We are not using the lower vibrations of red and orange as often. It is also interesting to note that in healing the chakras, the one which needs the greatest healing at this time is the Solar Plexus. This chakra resonates with yellow and lime green and deals with issues of personal power, self-worth, and confidence. In acupuncture the Solar Plexus represents the fire element and relates, at a psychological level, to healing the wounds of an unloved childhood. As we grow in spiritual consciousness, we lay the past to rest and move forward in life. We know who we are and what our value is. On a universal level, working with this chakra is about transforming power into love. This comes when we kindle the flame of love within ourselves. In terms of color, this means we are moving from the brilliance of the yellow light to the neutral and soothing color of green, a color associated with the Heart Chakra, the center of love.

Measuring the Electromagnetic Scale

The electromagnetic scale is measured in meters. Some of the waves, such as radio waves, are hundred of meters long. Others, such as the rays of visible light, are much shorter, about 0.0000005 meters in length. A wave of energy is like a rope which is oscillating up and down. The vibrations of energy are perpendicular to the direction of propagation. The wavelengths of energy are the distance the wave travels in one cycle of vibration, between two crests or troughs. The frequency is the number of waves passing a point in one second. The energy, or brightness, of a wave of light is proportional to the amplitude from the crest or trough to a zero, or center line. White light is a mixture of many wavelengths.

As we work with the vibratory frequency and oscillation of the energy waves, it is apparent that substances fall within the vibration of specific colors. For instance, Antimony and Berberis both fall into the yellow vibration. Though one is a mineral and the other is a plant, they share the vibrational frequency of yellow, and the symptoms they address when used as remedies share a psychological and physiological pattern. The mineral would have a deeper and longer effect than the plant. However, they would both help bring harmony to the mind/body/spirit, or economy, by virtue of their similar vibratory frequencies. How colors resonate in our body at specific frequencies is discussed in the section on chakras.

Chakras and the Human Energy System

Chakra means "wheel of light," and is a Sanskrit word that describes vortices of energy which filter vital life energy throughout the organism of all living forms. They function in all life forms and act as conductors for earth energy and cosmic energy. They act as conduits for the electric-magnetic force fields and stimulate and balance our life energy. The Human Energy System, at this stage in our evolution, possesses eight major chakras and twenty-one minor chakras. (All the acupuncture points are miniature chakras.) These chakras, or energy centers, filter energy into the ductless glands of the body and stimulate hormonal secretions essential for the growth, development, and balance of the body/mind/spirit. The chakras are also located in the region of their corresponding glands. For instance, the Brow Chakra is located in the area of the pituitary gland; the Throat Chakra is located in the throat near the thyroid gland. They are nonanatomical in character and exist in the subtle realm of the energy surrounding the body.

The chakras also correspond to specific colors that resonate with them at the same energetic frequency. They also correspond to sounds, have their own shapes, corresponding psychological archetypes, and emotional issues. I feel that by focusing our understanding on the physical characteristics and the emotional issues surrounding a person's problems, we can help rebalance the energetic system more quickly and efficiently through balancing the chakras. Color healing is already used as a form of vibrational healing to help balance the energetic body of a person in distress and can help people resolve their emotional issues with greater clarity and ease.

For example, if a person suffers from lack of confidence, a Solar Plexus issue, we could use yellow to help stimulate the center and give the vibrational energy of confidence and self-esteem. This works in a similar way to acupuncture, which stimulates the points on a particular meridian to give increased charge to the area deficient in energy. When the area is stimulated, psychological and emotional effects are apparent.

The color yellow, in all its various shades, is linked with the Solar Plexus. It helps stimulate a healthy function of this chakra and can boost a person's sense of value and worth. Conversely, when people are too deeply steeped in issues of personal power, also a function of the Solar Plexus, they may surround themselves with too much yellow. You may notice they will wear it, paint their favorite rooms that color, and even drive a car that color. They need a complementary color to bring balance into their lives. Too much yellow means too much ego. The complement of yellow is violet, the color of spirituality. This may be needed to offset the temporal desire for power. If you look at nature, you will see that yellow blossoms are always offset with violet and purple.

The Eight Chakras

Our Human Energy System has eight chakras. In this book the chakras are called by their English names and correspond to the location they have on the physical body. They traditionally have Sanskrit names which may be difficult to remember, though their meaning and purpose is beautifully described in Sanskrit. For instance, the Sacral Chakra is called *Svatistana* in Sanskrit and means "my own sweet abode."

They also relate to traditional Hindi folklore which correspond to each chakra. For those who wish to make a more in-depth study of these archetypal centers and the ancient myths surrounding them, great knowledge and understanding of how the ancients saw the function of each center can be attained. This information can be found in the bibliography in the back of the book.

I have taken the quintessential archetypal qualities of each chakra and related them to physical problems and emotional issues. These energy centers can be treated by using homeopathic remedies, color remedies, or flower essences. Blocked energy can also be shifted by chakra massage, meditation, and appropriate affirmations. It is important to know that there are many ways of shifting congested energy. We seek ways that offer deep-acting transformation. I have found the homeopathic color remedies to be generally effective in establishing balance and harmony in the Human Energy System. They are safe, gentle, and effective in the same way that homeopathy is.

What Is a Chakra?

Chakras are formed of subtle etheric energy. Their function is to filter energy throughout the body, from the most substantial form of life energy needed for our everyday survival to more refined levels of mental or spiritual energy. Chakras are formed, healed, or destroyed through the life force which acts on behalf of our conscious intention. They can be altered through thought, movement, and touch faster than by any other means. However, sustaining the high vibration necessary to change old existing attitudes or patterns of thought is not an easy task for most people. Remedies, color, and essences offer us a useful way of dealing with problems as they become present in our energy centers.

Color remedies increase the power and energy of a chakra and help it regain cohesion and function if there has been weakness or trauma. When color is homeopathically potentized, it acts as an energetic stimulant to the chakra and helps it regain balance and harmony. Since it is pure energy, it is also easily assimilated into the energetic system by the chakra itself. When a chakra is overcharged and drains energy from other centers, then the complementary color is indicated. This balances the chakra and provides an energy source for the weaker chakras to use so that balance can be restored in the system.

Using color remedies helps a patient resolve physical problems and emotional/mental issues without great struggle or despair. Balance is experienced as well-being, inner harmony, and, what in homeopathy is called, "being well in oneself."

Specific Cases for Using Color Remedies

There are times when a chakra may be damaged and needs stimulation from a color remedy to help with its economy. For instance, if there have been birth complications and the baby did not receive sufficient oxygen, you will see physical symptoms such as idiocy, blindness, and impaired sensory and motor function. This means that the higher chakras, which provide intellectual and spiritual energy, are also impaired. Using color from an early age can help the child overcome her/his handicaps. Color can stimulate the energetic centers and help repair damage. Where there is permanent physical damage, the chakras can still be stimulated to develop, and inner growth and development can proceed.

Although a child may be physically blind, it doesn't mean that s/he has to suffer emotional or spiritual blindness. Color can be used to stimulate the subtle body to develop even though physical damage is irrevocable. Our organs have inner or spiritual functions as well as physical counterparts, and using color is a way to build a strong inner or spiritual body. This has proven to be effective in the treatment of physically handicapped adolescents and autistic adults.

There are subtle ways in which potentized color can nourish the refined energy of the higher chakras around the sensorium and the glands related to them. It can nourish deprived areas of the brain and help with glandular function, motor development, and emotional and spiritual insight. Color remedies have been used with a sufficient number of people with physical impairments, and the results over time have been beneficial, strengthening, and vitalizing.

Color is a very gentle and safe way of stimulating energy centers. Recently, I treated a baby born without a thyroid gland. She is on thyroxin and homeopathic Thyroidium as well as Baryta Carbonicum. She has responded well to Turquoise 3x repeated daily over a period of months. She communicated in an interesting way. She used to cry loudly and with great force when she wanted feeding or attention. After the Turquoise she became less aggressive in her communication. She cried of course, but in a different way with less of a sense of desperation. In a sense, it was apparent she was confident of getting what she wanted. It didn't take all her energy to communicate her needs. She became more confident that her needs could be met. After the remedy she had extra energy for playing and was more open and direct in her communication with people around her. The color has strengthened something in her life force which was subtle but impaired.

Another case is that of an adolescent girl with congenitally weakened kidneys. She was sexually abused as a child and was given repeated doses of antibiotics for relief of kidney infections. Her kidneys were weakened from overuse of drugs, and she still suffers from chronic cystitis. She has responded well to both Staphisagria 200 and Berberis tincture. She was also given Orange 6x to take when she felt low on energy. This gave her strength and a renewed sense of vitality. I also feel it had a direct effect on her kidneys. She has had no further infections nor any reported cases of cystitis since taking the Orange, symptoms which she would occasionally have while on the homeopathic remedies alone. The Sacral Chakra, whose color is Orange, feeds energy into the adrenal cortex of the kidneys. It governs how we respond to sexuality, finances, pleasure, and issues of well-being. As she has improved in her physical health she has also undergone a shift in the way she responds to men. She is not as eager to give herself to anyone who shows an interest in her. She is more discerning. Her pathology, at an emotional and physical level, has been transformed.

In the treatment of a 29-year-old man with cerebral palsy who could not speak, or walk without crutches, and who had suffered abuse in care for most of his life, we saw remarkable changes while on Orange, Green, and Pink.

The Orange worked on his physical vitality, and the Green and Pink helped his heart. He wanted to die when the case was first taken. Since treatment, he no longer speaks of death, and he has straightened his spine, relaxed the tension in his feet, grown 2 inches, and is attempting to walk without crutches. Color had a profound effect on his gray and bleak outlook.

Understanding how the chakras work can help us find the suitable remedy for people. The truth is, it is in the energetic system where balance and harmony can help restore physical and psychological function. Using the

The Chakras	Location
The Root Chakra	located at the base of the spine in the perineum
The Sacral Chakra	located two inches below the navel and two inches into the body
The Solar Plexus	located at the nerve ganglion under sternum and over the stomach area
The Heart Chakra	located over the chest slightly to right of center to balance the physical heart
The Throat Chakra	located in and over the throat area and includes the mouth, jaw, and ears
The Brow Chakra	located over the pituitary gland between the brows
The Crown Chakra	located at the crown of the skull
The Alta Major Chakra	located about ten inches above the crown of the head

homeopathic colors in an appropriate way allows healing to happen at subtle levels, as well as in the more obvious physical areas of life. When we see regained function at one level then the tendency for an energetic leak is diminished at another level. I see this time and time again both with traditional homeopathic treatment and with the color remedies. Remedies heal what is subtle and intangible. We experience balance as well-being and right action. People can then move into more creative and healthy development when their energy is whole and flowing in the proper channels.

Color	Gland	Life Issues
Red	adrenal cortex	survival, grounding, organization
Orange	ovaries and testes	pleasure, sexuality, abundance, well-being
Yellow	pancreas	worth, esteem, confidence, personal power, freedom of choice
Green and Pink	thymus	community, nature, love, family, friendship, purity, innocence
Turquoise	thyroid	truth, will power, creativity, self-expression
Indigo	pituitary	wisdom, knowledge, imagination, intuition, discernment
Violet	pineal	beauty, harmony, spirituality, love of God
Magenta	pineal	pre-incarnation contracts, the collective unconscious, highest levels of creativity

How the Chakras Function
Following the Flow of Energy through the Chakras
Energy enters the chakras by passing into the subtle body from both the cosmos and the earth. Where earth and cosmic forces converge, the vortex of energy we know as a chakra forms. It is important to remember that this is happening in a dynamic flow which is constant and unceasing as long as physical life persists. Energy is being filtered in and out of all the centers simultaneously. A block in one chakra, which we might call a limited pattern of experience or arrested development, will limit the flow of energy moving in both directions, and will affect all the other chakras. If, for instance, there is an excessive amount of energy flowing in and through the Solar Plexus, there will be a weakening in the higher and lower centers. The ego will be strong but may base its sense of worth on what it has materially (the Sacral Chakra), and the Heart Chakra (or love center) would also be weak. Relationships were not always based on love but may have been based more on power. This would manifest in a person who tries to be more than s/he actually is; a person who focuses on issues of personal power and manipulation.

People blocked at the Throat Chakra would have an overly full Heart Chakra and a weak Brow Chakra. This could manifest as their inability to express their personal feelings, have limited ideas about themselves, and be unable to think wisely about who they are and what they are doing in life. This is often the energetic pattern found in creative people and many healers.

The flow of energy to the physical body is limited when it is blocked in the chakra. As energy flows into the chakra, it stimulates the ductless glands associated with it. The stimulation of the gland releases hormones into the bloodstream. This, in turn, affects the organs and tissues, stabilizes the emotions, and helps, ultimately, to fulfill the divine potential of each individual. Chakras, like homeopathic remedies, have a broad spectrum function which spans the breadth of physical and emotional development to the depths of karmic unfoldment and spiritual growth. When we add color to a chakra, we increase the intensity of vibration in that center. This has a potentiating effect on its function and flow.

Each chakra has its own particular function in regulating the glands and organs in its domain of influence. Chakras exist in the part of the subtle body known as the etheric body. This rests closest to the physical body and feeds energy into the body through nonanatomical nerves known as Nadis in yoga practice. These energize the glands. A chakra draws on the energy of other chakras to supply additional energy if there has been damage or blockage of function.

When a person is in the midst of emotional separation from her/his partner, the Heart Chakra would be weakened. We may call this energetic starvation grief or a broken heart. The Heart Chakra becomes dysfunctional as love ceases to sustain this person's life. The Solar Plexus Chakra then takes over temporarily to help this person build her/his confidence and regain a sense of personal power and self-worth. When this has been effective the Heart center, which has had time to heal again, becomes capable of functioning. In energetic terms this means the person is able to give and receive love again. It is usually at this point that another relationship appears in a person's life, or she/he focuses on more transpersonal involvement which engages the heart center.

It is dysfunctional for one energy center to do the work of another center. It is not appropriate, for instance, that personal power replace our need for well-being and pleasure. Feelings of worth, building of personal power, confidence, and freedom of choice are Solar Plexus functions. Pleasure, sexual enjoyment, the capacity for well-being, and the cultivation of abundance are Sacral Chakra functions. Just as in life there are boundaries which serve to enhance social organization, so too in the human energy system, there are appropriate boundaries which differentiate one energetic function from another. Each chakra supplies energy for its own particular function. When that energy is blocked it will leach energy away from that area. Then systemic problems could be expected to arise. The physical pathology begins to reflect an over-function or under-function of energy.

For example, when a person uses her/his sexuality (a Sacral Chakra function) to enhance personal power (a Solar Plexus function), it reflects a deep dysfunction and eventually pathology of some sort would materialize, usually to the reproductive system. The person is using the energy of one chakra to replace the function of another weakened center. She/he would need more Orange to strengthen the sense of ease and enjoyment, and Yellow to strengthen the Solar Plexus and develop a healthy functioning sense of self.

People who are unable to express themselves appropriately (a Throat Chakra issue) may have a very strong or overcharged Heart Chakra. They may be healers, homeopaths, or performers. They use their heart to contain the love they find difficult to share verbally with others. They may tire easily and suffer from weak hearts in later years. They could use Turquoise to strengthen their Throat Chakra and Green and Pink to strengthen their Heart Chakra when they feel drained.

People who are confined to only one way of coping or operating in the world may need to examine what is blocked in their lives that creates an inflexible energy field and stifles their creativity. If identifying with a particular way of being, such as being a healer or homeopath, is our only way of engaging with the world, we need to see what other function is weakened and put some light (i.e., color) into that area of our lives. It is also possible that a thought form or attitude about joy, ease, pleasure, or creative expression needs to be transformed. This can be enhanced through the use of color remedies that make this task of transformation easier. Color helps replenish a low energy supply so that the work of reevaluating our lives is easier and more joyful.

Color and Attitude

Daily, we see people in our practices who are repeatedly under par. Often they are not doing what they want with their lives, and are afraid to explore what it is that would give them happiness and satisfaction. They are fixed in a pattern of limited beliefs about themselves. They are also fixed in an archetypal response to the world around them.

This block to growth and personal development can be seen in terms of their colors as well. Often you will hear people say that they will wear only a certain color, and they would never consider another. Or they will say they have anxiety or fear about a certain color; they may be phobic about it. This is an indication of blocked energy.

Sometimes exploring the attitudes and archetypes of the chakras opens up a realm of possibilities that can facilitate transformation in our way of being in the world. Using color remedies changes our vibrations that can bring healing to negative and outmoded attitudes and beliefs. A shift in our attitudes occurs that can effect a change in our feelings towards colors, sounds, and life in general.

Color Healing and Color Remedies

Color can be applied to the Human Energy System through the use of colored lights, clothing, or inner visualization techniques. Homeopathic color remedies appear to be able to directly influence the nature of the chakras, and give both stimulation and balance to the whole energetic system. Depending upon the potency of the color, it will have various effects on the chakra for different lengths of time. Low potencies will need to be repeated more often. Higher potencies will hold for longer.

Color remedies increase the flow of energy, physically, emotionally, and mentally during the time they are active. We have seen changes at a physical level where pathology has been reversed. We have also seen emotional shifts in people's attitudes to life where significant changes have occurred to their well-being and fulfillment.

We know, from the provings, that color remedies have a direct effect on temperature and fluid retention, release irritability and tranquility, facilitate the expression of emotions, enhance levels of confidence and self-worth, and influence feelings of love and hate. Depending on the potency used color remedies can stimulate levels of energy over a period of time sufficient to restore harmony in a person's life. We have seen it directly affect energy levels in people who were completely exhausted from chronic and terminal disease. When given the remedies, they made a remarkable shift on all levels of being.

One homeopath uses Orange 6x and Saccharine Officinallis 30x for deep depression in suicidal patients. This remedy revived the energy and spirit of these patients almost immediately. This has become a prescriptive formula for deeply depressed patients who were unable to make healthy decisions or positive moves in their lives, and whose energetic systems were nearly completely blocked.

Problems and the Subtle Energy System

It is vital for the practitioner to know that, when a patient complains about certain emotional or physical problems, she/he is alluding to an imbalance in the subtle energy system. As we look for the core of a problem, it may be worthwhile to consider looking at the emotional issues of each chakra to see where your patient fits. If we look at personal problems as an external causative factor in a patient's life, without seeing that each person creates their reality by virtue of their intention and attitude, we are doing them an injustice with regard to their inner development and growth. When we address the problems and address over-compensatory tendencies, we help people move on in their lives and make healthy decisions about where they want to go and what they hope to do to fulfill their highest potential. We are, in effect, serving their higher consciousness. It lightens the burden on a practitioner and gives the patient responsibility for their life when we go to the core of their problems and literally shine light on them. We act as facilitators when we show the patient where the blocks are and give the appropriate stimulation required to shift the balance between health and suffering.

The Emotional Issues Related to the Chakras and Color Remedies

Each chakra focuses on different levels of emotional expression, life issues, and stages of inner development. This provides us with a hierarchy of consciousness to evaluate physical capabilities, as well as emotional and spiritual growth. We can see the emergence of individuality in terms of personal empowerment, sustained physical vitality, and levels of personal responsibility. Chakras develop as life develops. The first three chakras are formed during the first eighteen years of life. If they remain underdeveloped at this point then certain work will need to be done to increase levels of vitality and personal empowerment. For instance, if the development of personal power is arrested, the person will have an imbalance in their Solar Plexus. We may see an apparent lack of confidence or self-esteem that, ideally, should have been formed in youth, but because of a lack of love or nurturing, remains weak. These people turn out to be victims of power or manipulation. This may be overtly evident in a weak or impaired personality. From their stories we can discern damage at this specific level. The person may be plagued with irrational fears, be afraid to express her/himself, or have phobias or obsessions that mask a fundamental weakness and lack of strength. The person may also be hateful or resentful, and her/his power could be blocked with these negative emotions. If this remains a chronic state, and the person is not allowed to break free of her/his limitations or constraints, s/he will fail to grow and develop. We will eventually see pathology express itself in an under-functioning digestion, a congested liver and the problems that brings with it, such as weak assimilation. We could see problems arise with the liver, the seat of anger, or in the gallbladder, where timidity about love is reflected and where frustration can fester and solidify into stones. If the problem is treated allopathically and steroids are administered, then an early death would be predictable as a person became less and less capable of harnessing the strength to deal with the world, both physically and psychically. They would not find the energy to face their emotional issues. The allopathic drugs create so much weakness that people are left bereft, weakened, and incapable of harnessing the strength they need to get on with their lives.

Of course, there are homeopathic remedies which address these problems and their pathology. There is also a direct correlation between the colors and the homeopathic remedies used. These can be found at the back of the book.

It is important, if we are looking at an energetic/emotional causative factor, that we are able to see where imbalance lies and how it can be redressed. If we only treat the patient without looking at the deeper, and underlying issues of imbalance, we are not helping our patients in the long run. We are merely providing a quick fix. We may even be suppressing their physical symptoms when we do not look more closely at the more serious emotional and mental issues.

In our example of the Solar Plexus imbalance, healing can be accomplished with psychological assistance that helps to build a strong chakra by reinforcing the ego. It can also be done energetically using color, which directly works to stimulate the Solar Plexus, and helps the flow of energy through the chakra and into the ductless gland of the pancreas. We have homeopathic remedies which will address the underlying weakness as well. Both color and other homeopathic remedies will stimulate digestion at both the physical and emotional levels. We have the choice to work at many levels to help the patient through his difficulties. However, the remedies have a parallel effect on the body/mind/spirit.

Balance will appear first at the mental and emotional level where we would hope to see patients gain greater self-confidence and faith in their ability to get on in life. They begin to live the kind of life they wish for. Healing would then move into the physical level, where the actual problems with which patients presented begin to disappear.

I have seen in the provings that the color remedies transform the energy of under-functioning or unbalanced chakras and help heal emotional as well as physical dysfunction. Throughout all the provings, statements such as "better able to cope" and "stronger in myself" were repeated. This signifies that the chakra is becoming more functional, and the person is able to process their energy better.

Emotions are not the only cause of physical distress, but they do play a very large part in the healing process. There are often things deeply rooted in our energetic economy which can be triggered by stress. These issues give us an opportunity to be self-affirming and positive in our lives. They strengthen us and give us a realistic sense of who we are and what we can cope with in life. Using the color remedies can assist people through difficult times and through changes where the emotions run high and are volatile.

Emotional Issues: Colors and Chakras

If people are ungrounded and disconnected with the realities of a material and physical life, this will be reflected in their energy system. This will show up as a lack of vital heat or red and orange light. They will be lacking some of the strong, vital energy of the lower chakras, and their related colors and energy field will appear depleted. Either they may shun these colors or have a strong desire for them because they are arrested at this energetic or vibrational level. Sometimes simply asking people which colors they like and dislike can help you determine which chakras are in need of treatment. You can check out the emotional issues of the chakras and see whether there is correspondence between their issues and the energy centers.

Healings can be administered in the form of a homeopathic color remedy. The potencies range from 3x to 30c. Depending upon the degree of disconnectedness and separation we see in the patient, the remedy may need to be repeated over a period of time. As the color is ingested into the system, it stimulates those centers where the color is needed. The energy of the color remedy will stimulate the function of that chakra. As the person becomes more balanced, she/he will need less stimulation or repeated doses of the color remedy. This is an indication that the remedy is working.

Some of the signs that the chakra has been stimulated will appear in the emotional behavior of the patient. They can show signs of irritation, anger, or frustration, or can suddenly appear more relaxed, at ease, or understanding. They can develop a stronger appetite for more earthy things such as food, exercise, sex, or material things.

If an ungrounded person, who had little interest in food, suddenly develops a strong appetite, it would be an indication that the color remedy is working, and they are becoming more earthed. Patience, order, stability, a concern for physical security, and a desire to make their dreams come true are also signs of grounding. These are aspects of the Root Chakra and are associated with a strong vital force. Anger could also be a symptom which would indicate grounding.

The issues of each chakra and color are given in the chart on pages 42-43. They help you see that, when a person is discussing specific issues, you can relate those issues to a specific chakra and color remedy. If, for example, a person is blocked in their self-expression, which relates to the Throat Chakra, then Turquoise is the color remedy needed. Grounding and survival, as well as family or tribal issues, are related to the Root Chakra and the color remedy Red.

When a person is tired and worn out, Orange is the color to consider. The therapeutics of this way of working are guided by the emotional issues, and the color is then administered accordingly. It is a simple and easy system to follow. It is neither complicated or complex. It does require, however, that the practitioner be attuned to the emotional reality of the patient. It moves beyond the general physical symptoms and becomes anchored in life issues and developmental stages in an individual's life.

We are constantly evolving. We can facilitate that process when we acknowledge our emotional truths and take responsibility for how things are in our life. If we suppress and deny, then we will become susceptible to physical pathology. When we are at the stage of physical illness, it is difficult to sort our emotions, which, by the time we are facing physical crisis, may be very confused and entangled.

When we see a patient trying to sort out the issues of life which are reflected in her/his everyday encounters, then we have the clues as to which color to administer. If a person is traumatized by encounters with strangers, or is afraid to embrace life, we are looking at Root Chakra dysfunction, even though this could appear as fear, which is a Solar Plexus issue. Red is the color of the Root Chakra and would be a good remedy to help ground the fears of this patient.

Two Patients with Similar Symptoms Needing Different Colors

A few years ago I had two patients appear on the same day with exactly the same symptoms. They both were complaining of stomach cramps. One woman was a spiritual devotee of an Indian guru. This man was the Master to whom she lived in total surrender. She abstained from many physical and material comforts. She was also unable to look after her physical needs properly. She lost things easily, and wasn't aware of her physical surroundings. She was ungrounded and required Red, the color of earth and physical reality. This was also the one color to which she was most adverse. She was given one dose of Red 30 and within minutes her cramps disappeared, and she appeared more connected to people and her environment. The lack of focus and the quality of disconnectedness were gone. Suddenly she was present and in her body. Within a few minutes she became angry and wept about the lack of warmth in her life.

Later that day, a young girl of seventeen complained of the same symptoms. She was in severe conflict with her mother, who was both mentally unbalanced and neglectful. This girl needed spiritual understanding in order to manage her situation. She was given Magenta 30. This is the color of the collective unconscious and spiritual acceptance. This girl needed a larger vision of her life in order to come to grips with her unpleasant situation. This remedy took all her physical complaints away, and she had a dream that night which helped her see her situation with her mother. Within weeks she went to live with her father and began to study and make plans for her life, which she had been unable to do while in constant conflict with her mother. She was later given a homeopathic remedy which was deeper-acting and addressed some of her other problems.

With these two patients, the colors were given according to the emotional and energetic needs of each individual. We also do this when we give a homeopathic remedy. We seldom determine treatments based on physical symptoms alone, and it is the same with the color remedies. We give what is needed at the deepest level. For all deep healing to occur we need to capture the essence of a person's inner reality.

The Chakras: Qualities and Colors
The Root Chakra

The primary quality of the Root Chakra is grounding, defined as a realistic way of engaging with the world. This means being able to cover the essentials of life through providing food, shelter, and having work that sustains oneself and one's family. Survival is the main issue of this chakra. It relates to one's place in family and community, as well as tribe and nation. It also relates to organizational skills that help bring order to one's life.

A prerequisite for grounding is the finer, more differentiated quality of patience. Patience is the ability to see projects and relationships through to their natural conclusion without becoming despondent or despairing, anxious or frustrated. This requires a strong sense of grounding and determination. People who are ungrounded are not patient. They become easily victimized and frustrated. They often give up on things without seeing them through.

A subsequent issue is the ability to create a wholesome structure for one's life that is meaningful and fulfilling so that life can unfold in healthy and creative ways. Another issue associated with the Root Chakra is stability. Constant dramas or crises in one's life help to deplete and drain one's vital energy. Security is also essential so that one feels safe and not threatened in any way. If a person has little or no security that life can unfold without harm, then a person will not thrive. Lastly, we ground our creative capacities in life through our ability to manifest one's dreams into reality. The trust and belief that we can manifest our dreams is a genuinely grounded aspect of the Root Chakra. Without this we have little control over our lives, nor do we feel a sense of mastery when goodness develops for us.

The function of the Root Chakra can become impaired whenever there is uprooting or drastic change in one's life. Dysfunction can also be the result of war, poverty, or disease. When homeopaths describe the roots of disease, they are referring to the genetic predisposition that governs how we react in stressful situations, and how our body reflects that stress in particular physical functions. For instance, if there has been a familial weakness in the area of the Solar Plexus, and people in your family had a tendency to ulcers or indigestion, then, when stress attacks your system, it will generally be reflected in this same weak area of your constitution. This is a function of the Root Chakra, the center where familial patterns are stored in the genetic material. If these root issues are not addressed, then a person will react to each apparent challenge as a threat to their existence and certain life situations will trigger our susceptibility and create imbalance. The miasmas of disease are reflected differently under stress. A person with a Psoric predisposition will be overwhelmed by struggle and conflict and want to give up. One with a Sycotic predisposition will want to conquer their environment and will run the risk of becoming ill from excess work. One with a Syphilitic predisposition will be unusually creative and then begin to destroy herself/himself or her/his attempts at success. A person with the Cancerous predisposition will design their lives so that they will be unfulfilled or unexpressed. Our predispositions also mean that certain types of situations will make us susceptible to imbalance. How we respond is governed by our miasmatic inheritance and our genetic predisposition. This is all stored in our roots and will determine how the Root Chakra functions. It stores our genetic inheritance and we draw upon our reserves of energy when we are caught up in life's changes. The Chinese say that ancestral Chi, or energy, is stored in the kidneys, and it is the adrenal cortex of the kidneys which is governed by the Root Chakra.

Whenever we fall into the chronic patterns of response which have accumulated over generations, we are reacting from our "roots." This can be both positive and negative. If, for instance, people find themselves victims of life, it may be necessary for them to harness their strength and reserves to create a new and better life. Overcoming fixed ideas and eliminating fears helps revitalize energy from the core. This core of vitality and strength goes beneath our primary responses and gives us the ability to build a structure, create security and stability, and patiently establish order in our lives again, allowing our dreams to begin to manifest. Basically, this grounding helps us to choose life and renew our commitment to continuous growth.

When we begin to draw on these qualities and make them a part of our consciousness, our whole energy level shifts to one of greater vitality, and our self-esteem and confidence increase. We find that not only do we feel grounded, but we are actually in a better position to manifest our talents and gifts than we were before the upsets or crises which changed our lives.

So many people are now thrust into the midst of change as old structures break down. Some have managed well and others have not. What qualities people draw upon to handle the changes in their lives often reflect their deepest attitudes about life. Resiliency and a gracious trust in the sweetness of life can make the difference between living a good life or one fraught with struggle. It really is a choice to look at life as a positive force and to grow through the issues our parents and ancestors may have had to face. The Root Chakra is also related to issues of family and tribe, and the attitudes which maintained their continuity. It is not related to higher consciousness as much as it is to survival patterns which kept the family alive.

Development in this chakra depends on how strongly a person believes in her/himself and their right to a good life. If negative ideas predominate in a person's psyche she/he will manifest a very low-level archetype of empowerment, vitality, and responsibility. They will have low reserves of vitality, a limited sense of responsibility for themselves, and a real lack of personal empowerment. We would see this type of person as one of life's victims.

All these issues are covered under the Root Chakra and the color red.

The Sacral Chakra

The qualities of the Sacral Chakra, which is located 2 inches below the navel and 2 inches into the pelvis, revolve around the issues of ease, pleasure, sexuality, creativity, and abundance. These issues relate to how well we live our physical lives, and how well we value ourselves as physical beings living on the material plane. The life issues here concern how we feel about ourselves and our relationship to our existence as vital, healthy, and physical beings entitled to pleasure, wealth, and abundance.

How well we look after our physical selves in terms of cleanliness, beauty, care, exercise, proper eating, rest, and relaxation are also reflected in this energy center. Our physical vitality levels and ability to move freely and joyfully are governed by this center. Pleasure is an issue and is reflected in the ways we open ourselves to joy, seek happiness, and maintain a standard of physical well-being. This chakra is best exemplified in the statues of the smiling Buddha, who sits with a large, open belly, delighted with the pleasure of life. That deep pleasure that comes when we laugh, have a good meal, or feel good in ourselves and with life, strengthens and fortifies this chakra. Pleasure is pro-life. It sustains us and recharges our vitality for the tasks of life. It stimulates expansion at every level.

How we view ourselves as sexual beings with a commitment to a healthy sexuality is mirrored in the strength and vitality of this center. Dysfunctional or disconnected sexuality can be an indication that this center is not fully balanced. Problems with fertility, menstrual pains, or problems with reproduction, including difficult births, suggest that there are ideas and attitudes which do not engender a healthy view about one's sexuality. Sexuality can be used as a way of gaining personal worth if a person doesn't feel validated by others. Other problems such as premature ejaculation, impotency, and low libido reflect an unbalanced Sacral Chakra.

In general, this center is universally dysfunctional. We see people's worth measured by their material wealth and what they have. This is another aspect of this chakra. At an energetic level a person is dependent on constantly recharging their Sacral Chakra energy and will repeatedly grasp more and more as a way of reaffirming their sense of inadequacy.

In essence, this center measures what is enough. Sexual excess or abstinence, spending too much money, harboring a sense of lack, even physical prowess stimulated by drugs, and thin, lifeless, anorexic bodies are all reflections of an unhealthy Sacral Chakra energy. There is an old Dutch expression which says "you can't get enough of what you don't really want." This is a good description of a dysfunctional Sacral Chakra.

Appetite is the sense controlled by this chakra, so eating disorders and greed are reflected in this center. Interestingly, the fluid balance of the body is controlled by this chakra. In homeopathy, we look at retentive emotions as a causative factor in fluid retention. Emotions are also governed by this center.

The concept of abundance is controlled by this center. There can be an overemphasis or an underemphasis on wealth and material possessions and the feeling that one is entitled to the goodness of life. When people's worth is measured by the car they drive, the number of sexual conquests they have, or the clothes that they wear, they are disassociated from their bodies, their true selves, and this center.

Many physical illnesses with fatigue and exhaustion respond well to stimulation with Orange. This is the color of this chakra and helps to regulate the hormonal flow or energy of this center. It can stabilize energy here and help ill people regain their energy and vitality.

When Orange color remedies are combined with Pink, a sense of well-being is stimulated, and a person feels that s/he isn't good enough. Pink is associated with mother love and, when used in combination with other remedies, brings order to this center where so many people are blocked trying to prove that they are good enough.

The Solar Plexus

The issues which revolve around this center all have to do with a sense of personal worth. When people acknowledge their self-worth, they begin to negotiate with the world as warriors rather than as servants. Self-worth, self-esteem, confidence, and personal power are all qualities that are associated with what we regard in homeopathy as a sense of personal identity. The stronger this sense of self, the more a person can take command of their life and make healthy choices for themselves.

When people make unhealthy choices for their lives and get caught in situations where they are enslaved, manipulated, treated badly, or abused, there is a lack of personal worth and confidence. When patients speak of situations where they do not have the ability to stand up for themselves or fight for their rights, we are looking at Solar Plexus issues.

This may be reflected on a physical level by problems with the gallbladder, liver, stomach, small intestines, and pancreas. Hyperacidity, ulcers, and digestive disorders are an indication that people are blocking feelings such as aggression. They are literally swallowing their feelings of anger or hostility and behaving like the archetype of the Servant.

Power issues are a part of this center's sphere of influence. This can mean either a disproportionate desire for power, or a lack of faith in one's personal ability to express power in life. This is a masculine energy field and, often, issues surrounding the father appear in the personal psychology of the patient. Either the father was too strong or not strong enough, and the patient will project her/his issues which center around the father into the world. This is often seen in conflicts with authority represented either by institutions or large organizations where a person's personal identity is relatively insignificant. This is the chakra of the Warrior archetype. How well we harness our personal power will be reflected in how well we value ourselves, esteem ourselves, and have confidence in our ability to negotiate for ourselves in the world, however large or small our world may appear to be.

Another issue of the Solar Plexus is freedom of choice, to choose what we want and how we want to do things in life. When patients have given over their power to choose, this is seen as a dysfunction of the Solar Plexus. Calling our power back from all the projections we have created is a way in which we strengthen ourselves.

Yellow is the color which can help shift the energy of these issues of self-worth, confidence, personal power, and freedom of choice. It represents the sun and helps our light to shine.

The Heart Chakra

This center is concerned with all aspects of love and joy. It works on two levels. On one level it is the heart protector which acts as a shield against the negative and hurtful. It relates on the physical plane to the pericardium. On the second level this shield protects the purity and innocence of our hearts from exposure to harsh or unloving experiences. The heart protector provides a shelter for the heart itself and sustains the core of our being from hurt and abuse. People whose heart protector is weak suffer constant invasion from unloving energy, which often threatens and weakens them.

The core energy of the heart protector is made from the fabric of our experiences of love, whether that is family love, friendship, partnerships, love of nature, animals, or life itself. All factors which contribute to our love of life strengthen the heart protector. It acts as a barrier to protect the purity of our spirit which rests in the center of our heart. When we experience things as heartfelt we refer to being touched by someone or something.

The innocence and purity of our spiritual and emotional heart makes us very vulnerable. That is why love can send us soaring to the heights or bring us down so low we ache with pain. When the heart has been closed emotionally pathology may form as a result. They say that, after a heart operation, the people who heal the most quickly are those that cry easily, releasing blocked emotions. The tears act to release pent-up emotional energy which has been locked in the heart for a long while.

The Heart Chakra opens when we begin to feel love and allow love to come into our lives. This love comes to us when we transcend our egos and give freely and generously.

We learn about love, both conditional and unconditional, from childhood, from family, from relatives. We also see it represented in our culture in films and on television. As we mature, we find higher levels of expressing and experiencing love. The expression of love may acquire a very different appearance than the one to which we are accustomed. Love of the heart transcends all barriers, including death. Love endures in our souls and leaves indelible marks which build our spirit and nourish our soul. Love heals us.

The colors of the Heart Chakra are Green, for peace and balance, and Pink, for universal mother love.

The Throat Chakra

The issues of the Throat Chakra center on our ability to communicate our needs and to be creative with our life energy. Matters of personal will power enter into this chakra as does our relationship with the truth. This chakra is vital to our ability to express our feelings; to find words which convey our heartfelt emotions as well as our ideas and thoughts about life.

Will power is an aspect of this chakra and expresses itself in our ability to control what passes through our mouth. At a physical level this applies to food, drink, smoke, and drugs. All these pass through the narrow opening of the throat and can aid the power of the will or destroy it. The use of bad language, cursing, and gossip also weaken this center.

The throat is meant to be a center of truth, in all regards. That concept applies not only to how we communicate to others but also to the truth of what we ingest and take in. The Throat Chakra controls the sense of hearing; so the ears can be affected. If we are slandering others or hearing nasty things said and not taking responsibility for ourselves, we weaken our systems, particularity the throat center. Speaking up for ourselves strengthens this center.

How we use our will power directly affects the Throat Chakra. When we take too much alcohol or smoke, we are weakening the power of the will to protect and fortify us. Eventually, if we persist in abusing our systems, we will find it increasingly more difficult to harness our will. We need will to develop our skills and manage our lives. A strongly developed will controls what goes into the body physically, and what comes out spiritually. This is reflected in what is said and communicated. A will that is too strong can suppress emotions, and we see this when the throat becomes congested and heartfelt feelings are "swallowed." The will can be so strong that it weakens other functions of the Throat Chakra. When it is balanced, there is space for feelings to be expressed, and for freedom of thought as well.

It is through the Throat Chakra that we are linked to a higher source of light and truth. This is the point from which we channel the Higher Self. That energy enters the back of the Throat Chakra and projects onto the front of the throat where communication is focused. How well we express our truth depends on how well developed our sense of integrity is. This aspect of the Throat Chakra is linked to the area of the mouth, the teeth, and the jaw. Problems in this area may be due to unresolved issues related to personal dependency, and an unwillingness to speak up for what we believe and what we care about.

Integrity is our ability to "walk our talk," as the Native Americans say. This means that we do what we agree to do and we keep our promises. Integrity means wholeness and refers to our ability to relate to the world from the place within where we are whole and complete. This is reflected in the timbre of our voice, as well as the words we speak. Walking your talk is the opposite of the Native American belief that white people speak with forked tongues, a reference to the historical period during which the Native Americans were manipulated and exploited. The Native Americans are a people who have strong Throat Chakras; a part of their initiation rites required hardships and challenges to strengthen their will.

In our culture, we see weakened throats, loose skin on the neck in young people, or swollen throats. Many afflictions of the throat suggest that truth has been diluted and the belief in one's integrity is less than it should be.

We are not a culture that sings, chants, or expresses itself vocally. We revere those arts in which people develop their creative skills through painting, sculpture, dance, and music. These are legitimate ways of using this center. These skills are valued more than a direct expression of human emotion.

Children who have been abused, people who have been taught not to speak their truth, or people who have taken many drugs over a prolonged period of time have very weakened Throat Chakras. It takes a strong act of will to control our negativity, express our thoughts and feelings from a place of personal power and responsibility, and ask for what we want and what we believe is ours. Proper communication skills, which allow us to be detached and, at the same time, say what is in our heart, need to be developed in order for this center to strengthen. One of the sentences I use in workshops to strengthen this center is to say to others and to yourself in front of a mirror the words: *"You are beautiful and*

I love you." These words cause such a degree of distress in most people that they are worth saying to begin the practice of clearing the congested energy of the Throat Chakra.

The color associated with the Throat Chakra is Turquoise. It will help strengthen this center and seal off energy which tends to dissipate as a result of blocked emotions.

The Brow Chakra

This center is located between the eyebrows and is known as the control center. It functions as an antenna for many people, allowing them to ascertain whether they are safe and to what degree they are accepted. This center develops early in a child's life if they have come under threat from angry or volatile parents. A normally developed Brow Chakra will develop in early adolescence and be fully functional by the time of the Saturn return, which happens at around age twenty-eight.

The Brow Chakra controls many vital functions and is our conscious link to our life choices, and how we use our bodies. The use of the imagination to visualize action and events helps us to make our dreams become reality. The intuitive function of the right brain allows us to know the truth about people and situations. It helps us develop wisdom from our life experience. Wisdom is this center's goal. Its function reflects our capacity to take wisdom from life and distill it into a meaningful code from which to live our lives. For example, when we are told that fire burns, we may have a need to test this reality by burning ourselves. However, once we have had the experience we assimilate the knowledge that fire burns. This is wisdom at a very basic level.

Our use of knowledge for living our lives effectively also contributes to a Brow Chakra that functions well. We need knowledge in order to move ahead in life. Discernment is also a function which helps us to pick and choose who and what is for our highest good and greatest joy.

These five qualities—imagination, intuition, discernment, knowledge, and wisdom—make the Brow Chakra the center of control for 90 percent of our vital functions. Those who have a highly developed center are able to master their lives more easily than those who are blocked at a lower level of empowerment. A weakened Solar Plexus drains energy from the Brow Chakra, so proving our worth stops us from using our higher creative powers for ourselves.

The Brow Chakra is the beginning of our spiritual path. From living within the influence of this chakra, we learn the universal laws which govern human interaction. From here we can direct our energy toward the development of a higher spiritual code by which to live and eventually move up to the Crown as the operating center of our lives.

Indigo blue is the color of the Brow Chakra. It is the color of detachment and is cool and remote. It is the color of universal healing.

The Crown Chakra

The Crown Chakra sits at the very top of the head. It governs our communion with a higher source of consciousness, and its function is to help us to find bliss, peace, and beauty in our lives. It governs our aesthetic sense and connects us to that place within ourselves where we can find tranquility and serenity. When the Crown Chakra is impaired, health problems such as epilepsy, brain tumors, strokes, and disjointed mental patterns are found. Whenever there are physical problems in the area of this chakra, issues about growth, maturity, and development arise. Many times the person with these problems may wish to remain in an undifferentiated state; not grow up or mature or take personal responsibility for themselves.

Meditation helps to stabilize this center. It is the center known as the "Thousand Petalled Lotus," and governs illumination and enlightenment, the goal of all spiritual quests. It is the center which controls clairvoyance, spiritual truths, and higher consciousness.

Violet is the color of the Crown Chakra. This color gives peace, acts as an antiseptic, and can help to control pain.

The Alta Major Chakra

This chakra sits a foot above the head and relates to our link to the collective unconscious. The Alta Major Chakra holds information about past and present incarnations, and the contractual agreements we made with our Higher Self before incarnation. Generally, this center is undeveloped in most people and will open up in the "New Age." It is our telepathic link to all knowledge and activity, and acts as a communication link which makes our ideas and thoughts interchangeable. It is the center for higher truths.

The color of this center is Magenta. This color gives spiritual understanding and a sense of creative purpose to our lives.

The Colors and Their Qualities

Red

Red is the color of the life force. It has the slowest vibration and most dense energy field of all colors. It also has the longest wavelength and the lowest energy level of all visible colors. It relates to the planet Saturn and governs our physical and material existence. It is the first color to intrude on the senses when one has been in a darkened space. It is believed, of all colors, babies see red first upon leaving the womb because it is a similar color to that which has surrounded them for many months. Red is the color which the human eye will see first in a series of other colors. That is why it is used in danger warnings and alert signals.

Red is also the color which has the greatest emotional impact of any color. It is the color of passion, lust, and violence. The physical effects from long exposure are said to quicken the heart rate, create a release of adrenaline into the bloodstream, and give a sense of warmth. Red intensifies the senses. People sitting under red light for more than a few minutes report a heavy, leaden feeling, irritation and anger, and a quickening of the pulse.

When things are painted red they appear nearer than they really are. It has the effect of making spaces appear smaller and more congested. It is a color which demands attention and says *"Here I am."* Its conspicuous power makes it the obvious color to choose for giving commands. It is used in military uniforms because it is felt that the color charges the blood and lends itself to courage. It is a color linked to combat, aggression, and a martial spirit.

Color has long been used in medical diagnosis and red suggests inflammation and describes a quality of disorganized blood, seen especially on the face when people are excited or frightened. Red is associated with blood and heat in the body. In China the word for blood is "bloodred." The first association with this color is that of our own blood.

Red is also the color which feeds and nourishes the blood. It is associated with the heart as well as with the core of our emotions. Generally, it is associated with the physical, carnal aspects of life. The emotions associated with red are the ones which raise our blood pressure: lust, passion, and rage.

The bond between earth, life, and red is found in every culture on our planet. The rituals involving blood, for both men and women, are found in all tribal society. The poet William Butler Yeats said that red was the color of magic in every country and has been so since the very earliest times. Red is synonymous with life.

Esoterically, red represents the final stage in alchemy before turning base lead to gold. It had great import to the old alchemists, who were the precursors to homeopaths. Anger is often thought to be the next step to enlightenment, so this association of the alchemist can also relate to the inner stages of awareness.

Red is associated with the mineral iron and can be given whenever there is a lack of iron in the blood. It is indicated for anemia or any immunodeficiency disease, whether it is given with colored lights or in potency. It works well when people need to be earthed; to come out of their thoughts and into their body and feelings.

When people are recovering from illness, or, when they have been uprooted from their ordinary life through loss, shock, or trauma, this color helps them regain their grounding. Red can stimulate a person's sense of her/his right to existence. It is also indicated whenever healthy boundaries have been violated. It enhances our sense of place and promotes the courage and passion we need in order to live a meaningful and fulfilling life. Red is one of the colors which suggests independence and freedom.

Red is the one color which stands for life. Tribesmen in Kenya drink the blood of their cattle for nourishment and strength. They honor the color red as the essence of life. Graves found in prehistoric sites in their part of Africa were painted with red ochre.

It is felt that primitive man could only see red, yellow, and black; the colors of warning. As we have evolved, the refinement of our ability to identify color has developed, but red remains the primary color which the eye distinguishes from all others.

Too much red has been known to raise blood pressure and create irritability and anger. We have an expression in English, "we are so angry we see red." This could be the result of elevated blood pressure which inflames the blood vessels of the eye and actually creates an optical response that appears red.

People who need this color are those who are infirmed and weak, low in life force, or so much in spirit that they are not "on the ground." It is a color with great vital force. It could be used homeopathically for people who have inflammations on the physical level or deep emotional suppression. Too much Red can create hemorrhage and an overflow of feeling and it is to be used cautiously.

When we are using homeopathic remedies such as Ferrum, Mecurius, or Cinnabaris, which is Merc. Sulph., we would *not* use Red, as these remedies contain large quantities of this color. The last is a red mineral which has all the characteristics of a person with an abundance of red in her/his energy field. Its picture contains violence and manipulation and reflects an emotional person who is suspicious and seeks to hold onto power. This remedy creates inflammation of the bones, burning pains, swollen glands which can inflame and indurate. Merc. Sulph. fears murder and being murdered, poverty, dirt, and ugliness. This reflects a deeply dysfunctional Root Chakra; an excess of red energy congested and blocked in the energy system. It would be best to use one of the higher colors to help decongest the red energy which needs to be transmuted. It is evident with Merc. Sulph. that, at a certain level, there is also an impaired Crown Chakra where spirituality is not being nurtured.

Wherever there is epilepsy, there is dysfunction in the Crown Chakra. This would also be an indication for Violet or Magenta. Magenta is a combination of both red and green and can be used wherever you think red would be appropriate, but without adding the high charge that this color has.

Red can also be considered when we use plant remedies, especially those that survive in winter and have a strong healing effect on the vital force, such as Hellaborus, Bryonia, and Arnica. These remedies have the quality of vitality needed to restore life. Carbo Vegetalis and Carbo Animalis also possess the red ray of energy and could be used in conjunction with Red to awaken, enliven, and restore lost vitality.

At the emotional level we would consider giving Red to someone who was not able to express their rage or anger. It would stimulate the reactive forces blocked or deeply suppressed in the psyche. It needs to be given with caution at this level, certainly above a 12c potency. We saw in the original provings that Orange could also stimulate the emotions to the point that one prover tried to stab her husband with a fork right before her period. Choose carefully, based on the type of personality that requires this color, and warn the person that s/he could become very irritable.

Those people who do not need red are those with an abundance of it in their systems. For instance, people with high blood pressure have too much red congested in their system. They are people deeply engaged with life. People who have strong tempers, are hot by nature, and who can turn violent and aggressive easily do not need this color. People who are anemic, distant from life, easily defeated, or detached and fragile, benefit from it. People suffering with immunodefficiency diseases do the best on it. These may be

HIV and AIDS patients. They could also be patients with Guillain Barre (ME) and post-viral syndrome.

Red has been used by pregnant women to help bring on the labor process. It is known in India that stimulating the Root Chakra will also help women through labor and ease their discomfort.

The homeopathic preparation of Red can stimulate the birth process and gently help bring new life into the world. Conversely, it is not a color given to anyone terminally ill and ready to pass over. The color they would need would be Green for peace, or Violet for spirituality.

Wherever people are slow to react to life or lack strength, Red is the color to consider. It can be given to elderly people in very low potency to help their vitality if they are weak or infirmed, and their vital forces are slow to reactivate. However, do consider that it is inappropriate for elderly people to be fully and passionately engaged with life. They are also finishing their affairs on earth and a color like Magenta would be more suitable to their needs. Magenta carries the vibrations of Red as well as Green, and gives energy to the heart as well as vitality.

Red is the color of the Root Chakra, which deals with survival, organization, and security. This center focuses on the emotional qualities of patience, stability, structure, security, and the ability to make our dreams come true. If a person is able to live sufficiently from this center s/he is ready to create the next level in life, a level which relates to pleasure, sexuality, financial abundance, and well-being.

Red can be used for:
Physical Problems
Poor circulation, constipation, piles, varicose veins, rectal and urinary troubles, problems with the feet, knees, legs, childbirth, anemia, weakness, slow recuperative ability, immunodeficiency diseases all respond to this color.
Contraindications: Red should not be used by people with high blood pressure or who are violent and aggressive by nature. Do not repeat too often. Keep the potency under 30c.

Emotional Issues
Red addresses lack of grounding, feeling disconnected from people and environment, or spaced-out, feeling detached from emotional expression, or those who have a lack of emotional reality. It can be used for unstable people who have no structure to their life; those who are unable to patiently await their good unfolding; people who have trouble settling in a place or those who are unable to see a horizon in their life. It can be used for deep depression, and anxiety about survival. It is good for suicidal tendencies.
Contraindications: Do not give to people with a history of violence.

Mental Issues
People absorbed in spiritual practices who do not think about the practical realities of life; people who are very detached and live in another sphere of reality; dreamers, and indolent people unable to work or support themselves respond to this color.
Contraindications: Do not give often to people who suppress rage and channel their feelings into rationality.

Spiritual Issues

Red can be used for those who are locked into giving their spiritual energy to others, and who do not feel they have a right to their own life; for people who are enslaved and unable to freely live their lives; and those in need of spiritual courage to make the next move in life.

It is also a remedy which could be used for abandoned babies who have been put up for adoption. Each patient I have treated who was adopted had serious issues with the Root Chakra. Red could help root them in their own life force more securely.

Essence

The quintessential quality of red is imploded, congested, or compacted energy. Red is hot. The energy of this color is contracted, full of vitality, but potentially explosive. It is intense, dense, and slow-moving. Red provides heat, shelter, strength, and nourishment. It relates to the Mother archetype and the life force found in blood. It expressly asks to be contained, held in, or held back. Think of the Victim archetype as having little or no red in their energy field.

Homeopathic Related Remedies

All the Ferrums contain the energy of red. It is also associated with Mercury, and Fluorine, which contain the red vibration. The plant remedies which have the red energy are Berberis, Arnica, Carbo Vegetalis, Carbo Animalis, Belladonna, and Nux Vomica. Scorpion is the red energy, as is Lachesis, the snake venoms, and the spider poisons as well.
Caution: Red is used in cases where the physical vitality is weakened. It can provoke rage and anger if these emotions have been deeply suppressed. It can bring out violence and

antisocial behavior in people who are already too hot emotionally. Use with care.

Cases

Case One—A man, age thirty-seven, had Epstein-Barr for three years and he was so weak he could not work full-time and had to go on welfare. He was better out of doors and in the country. He developed a strong desire (passion) for the land. He was treated with several homeopathic remedies for over a year that generally helped him. When he was given Red 12x three times daily for a month, his energy levels soared. He was able to start a new work project that allowed him to work from his home at his own hours. He had frequent relapses of Epstein-Barr, but revived each time he repeated Red.

Case Two—A woman, age fifty-seven, who worked long shifts as a nurse and looked after an aging mother, did well on Red 30c given as a single dose. She changed her work load and got help for her mother. She realized she was a slave to her fixed ideas about helping others.

Case Three—A woman, approximately fifty years old, with involuntary stools each time she urinates, is doing well on one 30c dose of Red a week. She has had several remedies which have not touched her problem. She considered surgery until trying Red, which alleviated all of her distressing symptoms.

Orange

This is the color of joy, creativity, and pleasure. It governs the Sacral Chakra, center of ease, movement, pleasure, sensuality and sexuality, well-being, and abundance. It is ruled by the archetype of the Empress/Emperor; those people who live abundantly in the material world and who enjoy the good things of life. This archetype is a metaphor for joyful experiences, as is this color.

This color and its archetype is associated with people who have a healthy appetite for life. Orange governs the appetite, as the advertising industry so cleverly knows. Observe the way in which cheap, junk food advertisements are done in orange print. They appeal to the hungry person on a subliminal level. Conversely, too much orange in the system reveals a sign of greed, an indication that a person feels that who s/he is and what s/he has is not enough. This manifests at a psychological level as wanting or needing more. This may manifest as more food, more experience, more sex, or more money.

Orange, in its various shades of coral, apricot, sienna, or umber, is the color for people who are enthusiastic about life and are eager to participate and engage with others. However, they sometimes need the higher colors to balance their appetites. Orange can combine with turquoise or pale blue to give a spiritual balance. Many churches throughout the world combine orange, or terracotta, and blue in their buildings. A sign of heaven and earth is symbolized in this combination of colors. It is the mixture of the physical and the spirit. You can often see this in jewelry from the Native Americans and Tibetans, who mix turquoise and carnelian or coral.

Orange is also the color of vitality and, in shades of pale orange and apricot, it represents the sensual side of our nature. Orange is a color which has only one negative association; it can represent excess or indulgence. It is, on the whole, a positive and vibrant color that lifts flagging energy and gives a bright, affirmative quality to those who wear it or use it in decoration. It is a warm color suggestive of the sensual side of our nature and addresses our love of pleasure.

In Europe, there was no word for orange until the Middle Ages when the fruit of the same name arrived from Arabia. Previously things that were orange were perceived as an aspect of red. For instance, red hair, red clay, even fire, which is distinctly orange, was called red. Although it was historically associated with red, it is physically linked more with yellow. We see this in the fire center or Solar Plexus, which is responsible for transmuting food into fuel for our body.

Yellow and orange share depth, intensity, and brightness as an aspect of their nature. In a psychological way, orange behaves like yellow. It is cheerful, expansive, rich, and extroverted. This suggests that a person who has the heat and warmth of orange about them would also be confident, powerful, and rich in self-worth and self-esteem.

Orange relates to the water element of the Sacral Chakra and is essential in regulating our emotions. A deficiency of orange in the Human Energy System is also linked with allergies. We have found in the proving that the craving for chocolate relates to emotional suppression and deep longing for love. This has been transformed when the homeopathic Orange is given.

Patients get a tremendous sense of joy and well-being from this color remedy. One prover said she laughed all day and she found herself giggling for no apparent reason. That is why it has been used so successfully for depressives and suicidal patients. Melissa Assilem has used this color successfully for patients who threatened suicide.

Orange energy is found in amber, citrine, quartz, and topaz, which is a Sanskrit word for fire. Many birds and mammals have orange coloring. It is also a color which is suggestive of food; many highly nutritious foods are orange. Not surprisingly, it is one of the most popular colors for kitchens. One of the provers felt like redecorating her kitchen while taking this color in remedy form. She wanted to paint her walls orange. Color analysts know that orange has a high success rate among decorators, especially for the kitchen. It was interesting that the prover confirmed the choice of orange as a suitable color for the pleasure of eating. It directly stimulates the Sacral Chakra, which has to do with appetite and our sense of taste. In fashion, it is in constant demand and found in different shades and hues all year long because it addresses our sensuality.

The color is also associated with the metals of copper, brass, and bronze. They all have a orange tinge to them. It stands for fecundity and, in the Middle Ages, it had a sexual connotation. In early bridal custom, brides were adorned in orange blossoms, which symbolized fertility.

Orange provides us with a vibration which can stimulate our sense of joy and enliven our physical vitality. It helps people who are deficient in sexual energy to regain a sense of pleasure. It is the color which nourishes and stimulates the sexual organs and the hormones related to them. You can think of using Orange as a remedy when people have depleted their sexual center from overuse. It is also useful when people have negative attitudes that inhibit their sexual function, or lack a sense of ease and joy in relation to their bodies. It relates directly to our sense of pleasure and well-being. It can be given as a tonic when vitality is low, especially after an illness. It should never be given at night because the energy of the color will keep people from relaxing into sleep.

It can be used to stimulate lazy bowels and to help relieve slow onset of the menses. It would not be suggested for women who have a tendency to flooding during menstruation. I would recommend it for girls with irregular periods, such as Pulsatilla types or Calcium Carbonicum constitutionals.

When it is mixed with Pink, it opens people to a sense of fun and enjoyment. Some of the Nitric Acid or Nitrogen patients, who have difficulty allowing themselves to feel joy, would benefit from using Orange and Pink in combination. When faced with a long and boring task, Pink 3x and Orange 12c in combination help to bring a sense of pleasure back into life. Again, do not give this at night as it causes sleep disturbance problems.

Since Orange governs the water element in the body, we see that it is an active diuretic and stimulates urination when given in potency. Provers repeatedly mentioned frequent urination and a need to cry over things which disturbed them. Water imbalance is directly related to suppressed emotions and Orange seems to activate the body's ability to release fluid and stimulate feelings. It is, however, much more gentle than the violent emotions of Red.

Orange is a very physical color and could be considered for infertility if a couple is having trouble conceiving a child.

It is life-enhancing and life-promoting. It is suggested that it be used around the time of ovulation and given approximately 5 times daily for five days.

It can cause some emotional upsets and displays of anger if used too frequently, especially by people whose tempers run high and who anger quickly. In the provings, we have seen that people enjoyed being social more than usual, and were more friendly than usual while taking this color. A high sociability factor fits closely with the archetype of the Empress/Emperor, which represents the qualities of the Sacral Chakra when it is functioning properly. Orange can help shy people overcome their sense of reclusivity. It is the color which re-animates joy and well-being.

Orange can be used for:
Physical Problems
Consider Orange for bowel problems, infertility, period irregularity, slow onset of menstruation, anorexia, appetite disorders; when people have little or no appetite or when they have food cravings for chocolate and sweets. It is good for people who have post-viral conditions and have difficulty reviving their natural vitality after an illness. It is good for postoperative recovery and after dentistry, emotional shock, or trauma. It would be excellent in menopause, ME, Multiple Sclerosis (MS), and other autoimmune diseases.
Contraindications: Orange should not be used on people who have an excess of anger or rage. It would not suit the nature of someone with an abundance of energy as s/he may have trouble resting or finding quiet space. It could overstimulate their vitality and lead to restlessness. It should not be given at night.

Emotional Issues

This color suits people who are low emotionally. It has been used successfully along with Saccharine Officianalis to help people who feel suicidal. It has been used on its own for depression and emotional "funk"; where the feelings are blocked at a subconscious level and need reanimating. It brings people into the present if they tend to feel "spacey," and allows them to refocus their awareness into their physical body. It helps people connect with their sexuality and desire for pleasure. It is known as the "laughing color," as the provers found themselves happy and laughing much more than usual. They also cried more while on the remedy, releasing pent-up feelings which had been dormant. The crying was positive and released a flood of emotions. All provers said that their sense of well-being was increased while on the color.

Contraindications: Orange should not be used by hyperactive people, nor should it be used at night.

Mental Issues

This remedy is suited for anyone lacking a sense of their own well-being. It offers people who have a negative attitude towards their bodies and sexuality an opportunity to open up and develop a healthy degree of self-acceptance. It brings an awareness of the nature of pleasure. It stimulates appetite for the good things in life and increases an interest in sexuality as well as a desire for abundance. It can also stimulate a sense of creativity, playfulness, and fun.

Contraindications: Orange is not to be used by people who are persistently restless or anxious, nor should it be used at night.

Essence

The essence of Orange is a joyful, very physical state of being which nurtures life and its pleasurable aspects. It is the color of joy, health, and vitality. It can bring us into the present if we are locked up with excessive intellectualization and not in our bodies. It can help us to feel emotional if we are cut off from our feelings, and it can help release negativity and feelings of despair.

Homeopathic Related Remedies

Remedies such as Berberis, Calendula, Bellis Perenis, Rhus Tox, and Ruta fit the vibration of Orange. The minerals which correspond to Orange are all the Ferrum series, Beryllium, Selenium, and Tungsten. These are remedies which give strength and vitality and resonate with the qualities of Orange. The Natrums also have an affinity for Orange because they control the retention of fluid and emotion. Natrum types would benefit from doses of Orange. People living in Natrum climates, such as Northern Europe and Britain, where the weather is damp, would feel revitalized with occasional doses of Orange.

Yellow

Yellow contains more light than any other color in the visible spectrum. It is associated with the sun and with the metal gold. It is a diffuse energy and can create confusion when one is overexposed to it because of its lack of boundaries. Because there is so much light within this color, we can become disoriented and "spaced out" easily. It is also a warm color and gives off heat, though it is less intense than orange or red. Yellow lifts the spirits and gives people a sense of ease and lightness. People respond to it in a positive manner. It represents hope.

Yellow is a primary color and cannot be made by mixing it with other colors. For instance, orange is a combination of yellow and red; green is a combination of yellow and blue. Yellow is the color most closely associated with light and bright spirits than any other color.

Yellow is the color most easily associated with our personal power and prowess. Through its association with gold, it is linked with worth and value. It is the color of the Solar Plexus, the chakra which represents our sense of self-worth, self-esteem, confidence, personal power, and freedom of choice.

Yellow is the color of many body secretions and also the color of many foods and vitamins we ingest, which suggests the presence of sulphur. It is also the color which directly affects our digestion. It works to stimulate the stomach, pancreas, liver, and gallbladder. Too much yellow in our systems produces jaundice; an over-secretion of bilirubin, which signifies a weakened liver. Too little yellow in our systems suggests that we are not assimilating our nutrients properly, and we may have problems with absorption. This can also relate to how well we digest our emotional experiences.

Yellow is associated with the fire energy required for proper absorption of nutrients and is linked with the fire element in our systems. Like the sun, the color yellow implies that, when we are well in ourselves, we, too, shine and our systems function well. Physically and psychologically, the ability to digest our nutrients and our life experiences defines our state of health.

At a more esoteric level, yellow is the color of self-worth. This is reflected in our confidence levels and the ways in which we value ourselves in relationships with others. Our self-esteem and personal power show that we know who we are and what we want from life. The archetype which best represents these qualities is the Warrior. The dysfunctional archetype, with a diminished sense of self and weak levels of personal power, is the Servant. The association of yellow implies that this color represents aspects of the ego. Too much of it and we have an overly developed ego; too little and we have a coward, or as the slang implies, a "yellow belly." From time to time we may need a hero's dose of courage. Yellow can provide the energy for that.

Yellow is the color that lights up a drab and dull environment. It can bring a sense of radiance to clothing or a dull wardrobe. Too much yellow in clothing or decoration suggests that a person is overly concerned with power. There are new shades of yellow, recently developed by the automobile manufacturer BMW, that are suggestive of power and prowess on the road. They have names like Dakar Yellow and are reminiscent of endurance rallies.

Yellow, when it is mixed with other colors, is a metaphor for pain and for healing. When it is mixed with black, it suggests the sting of the wasp; when mixed with turquoise it represents the second ray of healing. When mixed with indigo it represents the colors of personal integrity. Yellow goes well with nearly every other color and represents a code of the self mixed with other vibrations of being.

Yellow is the symbol for enlightenment because it is the color that contains the most light. It represents the intellect, or the brighter part of the mind. As a color it has the highest reflectivity of all colors and appears to radiate outwards, or to advance. It is one of the hues which is brightest when fully saturated, whereas other colors will darken with an addition of light.

Yellow exemplifies the character of spring and the hope of warmth to come. Most early spring flowers are yellow, such as daffodils, crocuses, primroses, forsythia, and winter jasmine.

In food, yellow signals the presence of vitamin A and C. Different shades of yellow evoke either the astringency of lemons and citrus or the richness of butter and cheese. In nature, yellow is caused by carotenoids, and sometimes the presence of melanin.

In the animal world, yellow is worn as a color of warning. It is seen in tropical fish, insects, and exotic poisonous frogs. The subdued yellow of the big cats acts as a perfect camouflage for hiding in the tall parched grasses of the bush. Those animals, like the lion and tiger, who display yellow coats often have great presence and power.

In Chinese history, yellow was adapted in the early Sung dynasty as the Imperial color worn only by the Emperor, his retinue, or for imperial regalia. Buddhist monks wear yellow as a sign of humility. It is a color seen more in the Orient than in the West. It is forbidden to be worn by officials of the Catholic Church. Jews were forced to wear it during the Nazi reign of terror to set them apart from others. Yellow has also been used to describe cowardice among soldiers.

In the provings, Yellow showed a great affinity for people's fears and helped them over periods of doubt and worry. It was also effective in ending a bout of gallbladder colic in one prover who suffered for several days with distressing symptoms. It generally strengthened people who were low in self-esteem and helped others make clear and intelligent choices. All provers said it made them feel better about themselves and boosted their confidence. One prover became pregnant while on Yellow.

Yellow can be used for:
Physical Problems
Yellow relates to the organs of digestion and problems in this area, and is most suited for treatment of stomach, liver, gallbladder, and pancreas symptoms. It helps to decongest blocked energy and can be considered for any type of gastric colic. It is helpful for diabetes, stomach disease, hepatitis A and B, and cancer of the liver or any of the digestive organs. It has been known to work on gallbladder colic, taking away pain and congestion. It is an excellent remedy for any problems with assimilation, such as celiac disease, and can be used concurrently with other remedies that further enhance assimilation.

It is also useful for stimulating the right eye and improving eyesight. According to Chinese theory, the eyes are controlled by the liver. Provers noted improved vision and were able to read without glasses when on the remedy.

When the vital force is low, Yellow can help unblock congestion and shift energy. It is said to be extremely useful for colds and weakened lungs because it acts as an astringent and unblocks and decongests.

When there is an excess of yellow in the system it is wise to use the complementary colors of purple and violet. When new babies are born with weakened livers, and there is an excess of bilirubin in the blood, they are jaundiced. The standard treatment in hospital is to place them under ultraviolet light for a few hours every day to break up the congestion in the blood. Violet (in potency) should be used for this.

Contraindications: Yellow should be used as an astringent and a decongestant. It should be used in daytime only, as it can cause sleep disturbances.

Emotional Issues

Yellow is a color needed by anyone who has problems with confidence, lack of worth, low self-esteem, or a shaky sense of identity. It is particularly well-suited to those types of people who give their energy and life force over to others too easily and are too open in the Solar Plexus Chakra.

It strengthens the ego and helps people develop their individuality. Where there is emotional weakness or vulnerability, it stimulates confidence and encourages personal empowerment.

Contraindications: This color should not be used by people with an excessively developed ego, as it would increase their self-importance. It also should not be used at night.

Mental Issues

Yellow is the color of the lower, or gut level, intellect. This color stimulates the mind to help it become clear and focused. It helps to transfer "gut knowing," which comes from the Solar Plexus, to a higher mental level. Yellow can be used to help increase memory and thinking ability, and provides a rich potential for clarity and effectiveness.

Contraindication: Too much yellow can cause a dissociated feeling from an over-expansion of the mind.

Essence

The essence of yellow is its remarkable brightness and diffusion of energy. It is a radiant color and helps people to shine on an inner plane. It is a color which resembles gold on the material plane and, therefore, relates to earthly power and worth. On the spiritual plane, it represents lightness of mind, a willingness to transcend the limited ego and open to the power of a higher force. It helps people feel good about themselves and let their inner light shine forth.

Homeopathic Related Remedies

Many of our remedies which work on the issues of ego identification relate to yellow. It corresponds to Silica Arsenocosum Album, Sulphur, Fluoride, Antimony, Cadmium, Oxygen, Nitrogen, Helioantis, Bellis, Berberis, and Broom. Many of the plant remedies are yellow and work on digestion, assimilation, or repairing the digestive organs of the body. The other deep-acting remedies, such as Lycopodium and Chelidonium, work to create a strong ego function and address the problems of the liver as well.

Green

This color represents peace and balance. It is the most prevalent color in nature and soothes and comforts us when we are tired and weary. It is the neutral color in the visible spectrum of colors because it is neither hot nor cold. It sits in the middle of the spectrum and gives a respite from the heat of red, orange, and yellow and the chill of the blues, purples, and violets. It relates to our emotional balance and the healing power of nature. It corresponds to the Heart

Chakra and, therefore, is associated with the transpersonal issues of love, joy, peace, and unity. People who wear green often are those who are experiencing change and have a need for emotional balance in their lives. They can also be people who are resistant to change and seek the stability from this color.

There are, of course, many shades of green, each suggestive of a different aspect of the color. Most common is lime green, which still contains the fire of yellow; blue green, which carries the vibration and creative energy of turquoise; and forest green, which carries the energy of indigo and the stillness and detachment of that color.

There is also a toxic aspect to green which we find in poisons and mold. This color has a deadly, decaying quality to it. In the provings, this aspect of green was seen in the constant need to urinate that most provers had. It works as an excellent diuretic, eliminating toxins from the body. This aspect of green is part of its duality. It can bring us the positive energy which soothes and heals, and it can also bring us the disintegrating state of decay which helps new energy find its way into the system.

Green is the easiest color for the eye to see. The lens of the eye focuses green light almost exactly onto the retina. It is a tonic for the eye, which explains why eye shades and sunglasses use green tint to ease the glare of harsh light. Green has been used since ancient times as a respite for sore eyes. Medieval engravers kept a piece of green beryl to contemplate and relax their eyes after the intensity of their work. In ancient Egypt, the green stone malachite was crushed and made into an unguent to protect the eyes.

Green represents the emotion of love and is the color linked with the planet Venus, the planet associated with love and relationship. It was the color worn at medieval weddings to signify love, fidelity, and peace. It is the color which gives the mind and spirit peace and helps restore balance to ailing hearts.

Green is a natural detoxifying agent in the body and can help drain edematous tissue. It acts as a diuretic for congestive heart problems and has been used successfully with cardiac edema when given in potency.

It is also the color associated with decay, and plants do not grow well under green light; fluids drain out of them, they become lifeless, and begin to rot and decay. Green is associated with infection in the body, and, when this color is administered in potency, it drains the body of pus and poisons. When given during one woman's menstruation, she reported large clots discharged along with copious urination.

Green has this duplicity at both the physical and emotional levels. It is both the color of life and the color of decay. It is associated with nausea, poison, envy, and jealousy. It is also the color of rebirth in spring and eternal peace. Its dual nature is linked with its ability to fit both the top part of the visible spectrum and the bottom part. It is made from a mixture of yellow and blue and is known as a secondary color because it is made of two primary colors.

In the provings, it gave a deep sense of peace to people who were restless and out of sorts. It provided both relaxation and tranquility. People felt at ease in tense situations and felt that they need not hurry when taking it. It helped to relieve pain in the lumbar region of the back and behind the heart, and soothed fractious nerves when people felt agitated. Some provers reported restorative sleep, ease, and relaxation.

Its association with the Heart Chakra is linked to the issues of love, peace, and harmony. It works together with pink, combining natural tranquillity and motherly love. It represents the totality of love, care, and unity in our lives. Pink also represents a more global and universal quality of love which transcends the lower emotions of the three lower chakras. Love at this level becomes transpersonal and helps us to transcend the baser instincts. Green is an essential color in supporting life and can sustain us in our efforts to grow and be healthy. That is why it is recommended that we eat more green food.

Green can be used for:
Physical Problems

Green has been used successfully to drain excess fluid from the body. When there is edema, inflammation, or congestion, this color will remove fluid. It is best not to give Green at night because patients complain that they are up frequently to urinate. It has been useful for PMS (premenstrual syndrome) when women develop engorged breasts, have fluid retention in the ankles and belly, or when their emotions are charged.

It has helped when breasts become lumpy and eases pain in the left breast.

It has been used, along with other heart remedies, for congestive heart failure to tonify the heart and stop fluid retention. The relief given is quick, but not long-lasting.

It can be used for tired eyes and for headaches where there is a feeling of congestion. It can be used for inflammation of the testicles, or breasts, and for soft tissue swelling. *Contraindications:* If there has been a serious loss of fluid from diarrhea, vomiting, or kidney failure, Green would not be indicated. It should not be given at night.

Emotional Issues
This color has been used successfully on patients who have a serious lack of equilibrium in their emotional lives, who are barely managing to cope with problematic situations, where resources are drained, and they are tired and exhausted. It is especially good for people undergoing major life changes. Green helps to restore the balance emotionally and provides an opportunity to detach when feelings are running high.

It is good for fatigue and can be used whenever people are overly tired, overworked, and have trouble attaining a more peaceful state. It helps to restore peace and harmony to a stressed economy.
Contraindications: It should not be given to people who need stimulation, as it is more of a tranquilizer and sedative than a stimulator. It is not to be given late at night because it stimulates urination.

Mental Issues
Green is an excellent color for those who suffer from nervous tension. It is good for those who are highly strung and hysterical. Since it can soothe shattered nerves, it helps create a more balanced nervous system so that clear thinking and balance can occur. It gives a person a stronger sense of happiness and inner harmony.

Contraindications: Not to be given to indolent people who need their energy. Again, it is not indicated for night use because of the diuretic effect it has.

Essence

This is the color of balance and harmony. It can restore energy to those who are exhausted. It can help the body release fluid, which is another form of holding energy. It gives the heart a state of stability and eases distress and tension throughout the mind/body/spirit. Since it relates so closely to the Heart Chakra, it represents the qualities of love, friendship, family, unity, and joy, and can help when these areas of life become stressful.

Homeopathic Related Remedies

The remedies which correspond most accurately to green are Thuja, Craetegus, Cactus, China, Cuprum, and Chrome. Aurum relates to the heart as does Digitalis, Hydrastis, and Anacardium.

Turquoise

This is the color of creativity and self-expression. It is optically a mixture of green and indigo. It corresponds to the Throat Chakra and represents all forms of creative expression, communication, truth, and will power. It is the color first associated with spiritual values and healing. Many churches are painted terracotta and turquoise. The great mosque, Santa Sophia, in Istanbul, is made of thousands of tiny turquoise mosaics. The color addresses the spirit and is linked with the vast expanse of sea and sky which engenders a feeling of beauty, depth, and freedom. It is the color used most often in spiritual healing to soothe the soul. It is also the color most often chosen for clothing, decoration, and any place where beauty is expressed.

Turquoise is a color associated with the Virgin Mary. Her cloak was reputed to have been pale blue, and she is often depicted as the Queen of Heaven wearing her blue cloak.

Turquoise is represented by the Greek and Roman gods, Zeus and Jupiter. It is associated with spirituality for the Native Americans and Tibetans. Both cultures highly prize the stone of the same name and color, which is used frequently in their rituals. They say it represents heaven and earth in one substance. It is a color linked with royalty and from which the term "Blue Bloods" resulted.

Turquoise blue has a calming effect on the body and is said to be able to bring down high blood pressure. It is best used in rooms where people can relax.

It is associated with creativity and self-expression, so it is a color that would strengthen the Throat Chakra. It is the color which Native Americans feel nourishes the soul. When worn as an ornament, this stone is thought to enhance creativity, and promote healing to the throat.

In the provings, Turquoise appeared to have a definite link with excess catarrh, which diminished when Turquoise was taken. For example, a large, overweight woman began to lose weight while on the remedy. It may stimulate a sluggish thyroid gland.

It also shows a strong affinity for the mouth, which is governed by the Throat Chakra. One prover developed a tooth abscess while proving the remedy, which, in homeopathic terms, would suggest that it could heal this condition.

It could be considered for mouth ulcers, problems with the tongue and teeth, and an ulcerated throat.

At an emotional level Turquoise helps to increase communication and encourages people to say things they often found difficult or awkward to verbalize. It was used by musicians who reported that their music was more attuned and creative. It was given to a young baby born without a thyroid and, along with allopathic Thyroxin, homeopathic Thyroidium, and constitutional remedies, has strengthened her ability to communicate and to express what appears to be a very strong will.

Turquoise can be used for:
Physical Problems
The physical problems associated with turquoise relate to inflammation, particularly around the throat and mouth area. It will help a cold or sore throat clear up more quickly, and is good for underactive and overactive thyroid problems since it brings balance to this gland. It helps balance the thyroid and parathyroid.

It is used for problems of the teeth and gums and has been used successfully in alleviating toothache. It can be considered for mouth ulcers, ear infections, sore throat, and bronchial inflammations. It may be good for obesity where the thyroid is underactive and the patient has low energy, tires easily, and is apathetic.

Contraindications: Turquoise is not recommended for a person currently taking drugs or antibiotics. It would be best to wait for a few weeks until these drugs have left the system. It can be given both at night and during the day.

Emotional Issues

Where there are problems with self-expression this is an excellent color to use. It stimulates communication skills and strengthens a person's ability to speak up for her/himself. The throat is easily weakened with drugs, overeating, smoking, and drink; and this weakens the will. Any time the will needs to be engaged to achieve some task and is weak or shows decreased function, this is a color worth considering. For instance, if someone wants to quit smoking or wants to begin a diet, this would strengthen her/his resolve.

Turquoise strengthens the will and helps people resolve their personal addictions more easily. It has been seen to be effective where abuse has weakened a person's ability to speak out for her/himself. Musicians, artists, and people who are sensitive to the inner meaning of life have benefited from taking Turquoise. It helps people communicate their feelings or intentions. It is good for singers and people who overuse their throat.

Contraindications: It is not a substitute for communication but helps resolve tension in this sphere where it is blocked.

Mental Issues

The mental issues surrounding Turquoise relate to the ability to hear and express the truth. People may have resistance to speaking up for themselves and are afraid of repercussions. It may also affect those who have very fixed ideas and have trouble hearing the opinions or feelings of others. It works to strengthen the will so that clear intentionality can be expressed.

People who are very critical of others, who gossip and speak maliciously, could benefit from this color. Since so much negative energy is channeled through the throat, this color strengthens the throat and makes it less likely for energy to drain away and dissipate into negativity. For anyone who has problems differentiating the truth, this is also a good remedy.

Contraindications: None.

Essence

The essence of Turquoise is that it represents the truth; both the truth itself, and our personal expression of it. It stimulates our creativity and clears a path for us to express ourselves in the highest and most joyful ways. It helps define a person's individuality by strengthening their will. It works on the Throat Chakra and is associated with all the organs of speech, hearing, and ingestion.

Homeopathic Related Remedies

Turquoise relates to Aluminum, Stannum, Ignatia, Causticum, Aconite, Argentum, Tuberculinum, Beryllium, Lithium, Phosphorus, and Caladium as remedies.

Indigo

This color is cool or chilly. It symbolizes the intellect and emotional detachment. It corresponds to the Brow Chakra, or, what is known in yoga, as the control center of the body. This is the seat of the pituitary gland, which stimulates growth and controls reproductive cycles in the body. Indigo is a color of the mind and heals what is inflamed and impassioned.

Indigo acts as an anesthetic, and gives soothing and cooling relief from the pain of inflammation. It is known as the universal healing color. It suggests mental detachment and coolness of emotions. It is ethereal, more a color of the intellect than the passions.

The color has the ability to lower blood pressure, cool a fever, and give clarity and lucidity to the mind. It promotes detachment from overheated emotions. It is the color which is universally favored above all other colors. It is a favored color for fashion and decoration. Indigo is also the color most closely associated with the qualities of wisdom, discernment, knowledge, imagination, and intuition. These are the qualities of the Brow Chakra.

Indigo is the color of universal truth. It may be slightly cold, and a little merciless, but it is able to cleanse and calm the spirit. If Indigo is used too much, it has the ability to unground people and keep them fixed in the realm of the mind; they can live too much in their intellect and forget the physical realms of the body.

Indigo calms frayed nerves and anxious states. When people are too strongly engrossed or engaged in problems, this color can promote cool, unemotional mental powers and control. This can help people step back from a menacing situation.

For anyone suffering from depression, Indigo is not a suitable color. They need a color which reanimates their ability to feel, not one that detaches them from their feelings. The coolness of Indigo is suited to anyone who is too hot, too engaged, or too inflamed in their feelings and thoughts.

Indigo is used in color healing to tonify the lymph, and works especially on the mucous surfaces. It has a cooling quality which soothes and helps regenerate life energy. It can give a feeling of exhilaration to the mind and can increase physical strength as a result of this. It can act as a tonic for general health. Indigo is believed to be useful for congestive problems in the pelvis, and is even considered useful for sterility problems in both men and women. It is used for insanity, fever, and tuberculosis, and has been useful in the treatment of asthma, epilepsy, and chronic diseases where there has been degeneration.

At a psychological level, Indigo is used to cleanse and clear the psychic currents of the body. It can purify and stabilize fear and repressed feelings. It is associated with the pituitary gland, which sits behind the brow and is linked with the Brow Chakra. It stimulates the senses and can be used with dysfunction of the eyes, ears, and nose.

In the provings, it upset a woman who lead a very sedentary life. She worked in an office all day and was a very solitary person. The remedy caused her severe distress and unhappiness. The only thing which alleviated her suffering was to be massaged and cuddled. Indigo represents electron current flow and is connected with the electric end of the electromagnetic scale. Touch warms and is connected with magnetism, so it works on the opposite pole of the electromagnetic scale. This remedy was ultimately healing since it allowed her access to her deep needs. It helped her find her healing through human contact and warmth. It made her seek a solution to her sense of separation.

Indigo was also found to be useful to people who needed to use their minds to create healthy boundaries which protected them from invasive and intrusive people. It gave a clear mental framework and helped people resolve their emotional difficulties by thinking about their problems with greater clarity and in a more expanded way.

It helps clear headache, inflamed eyes, and soothes itchy scalp. It is best given at night or early in the morning and has a strong affinity to dawn and dusk when the sky is a beautiful shade of indigo.

While on the remedy, one of the provers found she became very chaotic and couldn't find obvious things she had left in front of her. She made writing mistakes and felt very disoriented for the first hour after taking the remedy. This suggests that it would be useful for dyslexia and confused states of mind. It also seemed to produce a clear picture of mental control, and those who took it in the provings felt they could control their lives with a greater degree of conscious mastery than before.

Indigo can be used for:
Physical Problems
The physical problems which Indigo addresses have been mentioned above. It acts as an anesthetic and can help relieve pain. It acts as a natural blood purifier and helps alleviate lymphatic congestion which causes inflammation. It can be used effectively for swollen joints, boils or carbuncles, skin irritation, or to soothe the internal organs.
Contraindications: None.

Emotional Issues
Indigo has a profound influence in this realm. It is good for anxiety and fearful states, or when the emotions run high. It cools, relaxes, and helps the emotions become detached. People find they are more analytical. It is good for an insane and agitated state.

Contraindications: It is not good for depressed states and can make a person more depressed and dissociated from her/his feelings and body.

Mental Issues

This color is very good for helping to organize thought and encourage economic thinking. It helps the mind focus and elucidate matters which weigh on the mind. It is a good tonic for tired and overused minds. It helps restore the balance where clarity has been lost.

Contraindications: It is not suitable for people who analyze constantly, and who are always in their heads. It would only accentuate that.

Essence

Indigo is a coolant and brings order to strongly heated and chaotic states, whether physical, emotional, or mental. It assists the conscious mind to maintain a state of control. It has a clear, soothing energy which can be utilized for consciousness and truth. It is the color of wisdom, truth, and integrity.

Homeopathic Related Remedies

Anterior and Posterior Pituitary, Sepia, Indigo, Lithium, Cobalt, Lachesis, Crotalus, Belladonna, Cuprum, Picric Acid, Phosphorus, and Camphor all relate to Indigo.

Violet

This color is associated with serenity, beauty, and spirituality. It works on the Crown Chakra, located at the top of the head, and helps establish the link between the personality, or smaller self, with the Source, also known as the Higher Self. It enhances our intimate relationship with our inner selves, the place of "peace beyond all peace." This is the place of inner stillness.

Violet can soothe and bring comfort, but also can act as an anesthetic and purifier on the physical level. Wherever there is violet, there is a strong link to the spiritual. It represents the color of the soul.

It is traditionally felt that violet represents the spiritual aspect and purple stands for the temporal element of power. Purple was a color reserved only for nobility both in Roman times and in Byzantium. It was very expensive to make and required the use of thousands of tiny mollusks to obtain the color. The expression, "to the purple born," comes from Byzantium, where all queens were required to give birth to future emperors in a room completely swathed in purple silk. This may have actually been quite hygienic, as purple and violet are both anesthetic in nature. Purple is now worn by high-ranking officials in the Catholic church at specific times during the liturgical year.

Violet is associated with the pineal gland, located in the top of the skull. Scientists are still baffled by the function of this gland. Esoteric healers and Oriental teachers share the belief that the function of the pineal gland is to open our spiritual center at the Crown Chakra. The pineal gland actually responds to light in a way similar to the eye. It is made of tiny rods and cones which are light-sensitive. It is felt that functions such as menstruation in women are controlled by the light sensitivity of this gland. Other pineal functions include our reaction to jet lag, fatigue associated with our intake of light, and the production of melatonin, a secretion of the pineal gland.

Tibetan lamas are known to practice specific yoga postures and say mudras and prayers which stimulate the pineal gland to secrete an essence they call nectar, a substance reputed to enhance feelings of ecstasy and bliss. This takes many years of devotion and practice to achieve.

Violet is found in nature in the beautiful flowers of spring and summer. It is seldom found in the animal kingdom, but in the mineral world can be found in manganese, magnesium, amethyst, and fluorine. It is found to enhance awareness when used in crystal healing and helps to open the spiritual centers more readily.

All the magnesium remedies work on the Crown Chakra and have a strong effect on inner stability, the alleviation of pain, and well-being. Problems with epilepsy, alcoholism, and nervous tension respond to this color whether it is given in remedy form, crystal healing, or color treatments.

Violet created an "otherworldly feeling" for many of the provers. It created nausea, disorientation, and headache in some provers, which means it would be useful in treating those conditions in ill people. It has been used to palliate pain and as a supplement to treat cancer of the pineal gland, giving relief and peace.

It was used on a highly evolved spiritual teacher in India who complained of chronic aching in his feet and legs. He was given Violet 6x in a split dose, and all of his pain disappeared. He resonated with the violet ray so strongly it seemed to be the best medicine to give him, and he was willing to try the treatment.

It has also been used by headache sufferers who were troubled by spiritual and ethical problems. These sufferers had conflicts between higher spiritual ideals and their emotions. Violet relieved the pain and the headaches never reappeared.

Violet is best used by the elderly, as it is a vibration to which they are more closely attuned. It is also good for those who have difficulty finding a spiritual path in life. This could help them attune to a greater understanding of their purpose in life, as well as help develop a more refined sense of beauty and serenity.

It has been used successfully to treat a patient who was both epileptic and alcoholic. Interestingly, he was an artist and was unable to see or paint violet or purple until he took the remedy. Whenever he attempted to paint these colors, they appeared as a muddy brown. After the remedy the color he painted was close to a natural violet.

It has been found that people lose their sense of ego identity when exposed to too much violet. If people are not grounded in their personal identity they easily become susceptible to the influence of others. They find it difficult to make decisions, be affirmative, and can become touchy and irritable. They can become too ungrounded in their spirituality. However, Violet is a gentle color and can give great comfort to those who suffer from too much sensitivity.

Violet can be used for:
Physical Problems
Violet light, because of its affinity to the Crown Chakra, can be used to help brain disorders such as alcoholism, epilepsy, and neurosis. It is particularly good for stopping pains and

could be used for menstrual cramps, headaches, and any pain around the head and shoulder area.

Contraindications: It is felt that, when people are too sensitive, Violet could make them uneasy and irritable. Magenta may have better results as it carries the red and green rays. It is suggested that if there is mental or emotional instability a small amount of Violet can be used, but, once the patient becomes restless or uneasy, it is best to stop. It is best given at night.

Emotional Issues

This color can be used to open up realms of spiritual understanding, ease the emotions, and bring the gift of peace and spiritual insight. It is known to soothe nervous conditions in which a person is fractious and out of sorts with her/himself. Violet can bring emotional stability to violent minds and relief to neurotic states of anxiety and chronic worry.

Contraindication: Use in limited dosage. Give the remedy and wait to see how the patient responds before giving a second dose of the remedy. Use caution with hypersensitive people.

Mental Issues

Violet gives a person a spiritual or higher outlook on life. It can also ease egotistical streaks in people. This can be useful for anyone trying to grow emotionally. At times, too strong an identification with the spiritual can limit the individuation, or healthy ego development, of a person, and if this is the case, be wary about giving it to people who need to get out into the world and live. Violet can make a person surrender their ego too readily. Finding a balance with this color is important.

Contraindications: Use judicially on people with weakened ego development. They can become very sensitized, even temporarily insane.

Essence

Violet is the color of our higher spiritual nature. It reflects the Divine light within us and helps us to connect to beauty around us and serenity inside ourselves. It is gentle and healing, and provides cleansing of the aura and attunement with the spiritual aspects of life.

Homeopathic Related Remedies

The Magnesiums all relate to the color violet, as does Manganeum. These remedies focus on the issues of the Crown Chakra. Hydrogen corresponds to the violet ray, as does DNA and other life-building substances. Iris Vericolor and Pansy also correspond to this color. Violet Fluorine, and Amethyst gem remedies also carry this vibration.

Pink

This is the color of universal mother love. It is often a favorite of young children and is a color associated with the Heart Chakra. It pertains to the purity and innocence of our hearts and helps open our capacity to give and receive love. It is a strong color often found in the aura of babies, and visible under Kirlian photography. It is the color which reflects the joy of life and is a muted shade of red.

Pink refers to rosiness and is an indication that there is vitality and life within us. Pink is often associated with little girls, but this is now changing as Pink is a color which suits many men and is finding its place into men's fashions. It is a color which is positive, loving, and a sign of purity and inno-cence. Pink represents joy and tenderness.

In the provings done on Pink, all provers had a dream associated with motherhood. They dreamed that either they were physically close to their mothers or were pregnant, were giving birth, or holding a baby. This was not specific to women; men also had dreams of being held by their mothers or loved and cherished by their mothers. Over six provers shared this dream about mother love and provided a strong indication for how it can best be used.

Pink is a color closely associated with gentleness, sweet-ness, and naiveté. It is a color also associated with youth and childhood. When it is worn or used in decoration, it is linked with the softer, sweeter side of life.

Pink, in the provings, made every one feel well. They found that their problems were less acute, and they could manage their problems better. They all reported feeling well in themselves. Even provers who had serious family, finan-cial, or health problems responded well while on the reme-dy. It did have a specific action on the physical body in the area of skin problems. It worked well with dry eczema, acne, and skin rash. These are also conditions, which, at an eso-teric level, are thought to be reflections of feeling unloved.

Pink can be used for:
Physical Conditions
Pink can be used for heart problems and is excellent for reviving vitality without the aggressive energy of Red or Orange. It can be used to help people overcome shock, such as the trauma of childbirth, injury, or grief. It is a general

toner and helps people through difficult times of change when they feel tired, fed up, or exhausted. It can be used for any skin condition which suggests a person may be somatizing feelings of rejection and feeling unloved.

Contraindications: None.

Emotional Issues

Pink is a color associated with love. Whenever there is a hardening or an emotional closing down, the color can be used to add a soft and gentle quality to a person's life. It is good for heartache, loss, and emotional suffering, especially in association with the loss of motherly or feminine love.

Contraindications: It is not just a woman's remedy. It can be given to either sex at any age, wherever there is loss of love or grief. When combined with Orange it adds vitality and a sense of joy to any situation.

Mental Issues:

Pink can be given to add an emotional element to the harsh light of the mind. It offers a sweetness and a refreshing quality to harsh mental activity.

Contraindications: None.

Essence

Pink is the color of love. It offers us the bloom of the rose, the sweetness of youth, and the joy of the heart. It suggests something childlike in us which relates to eternal youth, innocence, and mother.

Homeopathic Related Remedies

Ignatia, the Muriaticums, Kali Phos, Phos Ac., Pulsatilla, and Impatiens. The Milk remedies would also correspond to Pink as they promote self-love.

Magenta

This color represents the highest level of creativity and is associated with the collective unconscious. It is a mixture of green, red, and violet, and encompasses the energy of the life force heat of red, the peace, harmony, and neutrality of green, and the serenity of violet. It corresponds to the Alta Major Chakra, which sits about a foot above the Crown Chakra and is concerned with our higher purpose in life.

This chakra represents the collective unconscious and the bonds of humanity which make us all one. It is the color Rudolph Steiner believed stood for ultimate creative expression. It is a color reserved for special occasions and creative ventures. Whenever we want a depth of understanding which supports our deepest spiritual nature, Magenta is the color of choice.

It is used in color healing to stimulate the adrenals, the heart, and the sexuality of a person because it is made in part with red. It is said to strengthen the heart muscles and stabilize the heart rhythm. It has a diuretic effect as well because of the green component. It should be considered whenever there is fluid retention and also when the patient may need the extra vitality they receive from Red. It can be considered for elderly people as a tonic.

It stimulates sexuality by increasing the circulation and increasing the rate at which the heart pumps blood. Also, it is felt that many female disorders are due to an imbalance in Magenta. It could be used as a remedy for slow or late onset of the menses, infertility, endometriosis, or frigidity.

In the provings, Magenta helped people gain insight into their problems. It added a spiritual and realistic dimension to the way they viewed their problems, seemed to elevate those who were too grounded in their thinking, and ground those who were too "airy" in their approach to life.

It was given to a woman who developed weeping sores on both her legs at a crisis point in her thirty-year marriage. She had not responded to any other remedies. She felt that she could not see a future for herself if she stayed in the marriage, and she did not know what to do. This color helped her focus and gave her a horizon. When she took the remedy, her wounds began to heal and she found the sense of freedom she needed to begin to think about what she wanted from life.

It has been given to victims of abuse and to children who had neglectful parents. In all cases it helped the person reestablish links with her/his Higher Self and gain wisdom and insight.

The esoteric issues of the Alta Major Chakra correspond to the contracts made with our guardian spirits before incarnation. This color links us to the distant memory of past lives and also to the spiritual realm of guidance, protection, and purpose.

Magenta can be used for:
Physical Problems
It is good to use as a heart tonic. Also consider its use for impotency, frigidity, and low libido.
Contraindications: Magenta should not be used on hysterical patients.

Emotional Issues

Magenta is given when there is lack of insight, or when the emotions are too strongly engaged and an overview of the presenting problem is necessary. It suits people who have trouble envisioning a larger horizon in life.
Contraindications: None.

Mental Issues

Great thinkers gravitate to this color. It awakens latent creativity, and, at the same time, stimulates the sexual realms. This energy can be transmuted into creative expression through the use of this color. It elevates the thinking toward higher realms of awareness while maintaining a grounded and realistic approach to life.
Contraindications: None.

Essence

The essence of this color is creativity and insight. It combines the best of the vital force contained in the red with the peace and tranquility of green. It enhances our acceptance of what is universal in mankind. It stimulates our creative powers.

Homeopathic Related Remedies

Strontium, the Kalis, Manganese, Digitalis, Niobium, Molybdenum.

Spectrum

This is a combination of all the colors commonly known as rainbow. As a remedy, it has a very strong affinity to heal immuno-suppressive diseases or diseases that weaken the energetic system. It has been used successfully with ME,

AIDS, HIV, chronic fatigue syndrome (CFS), post-viral syndrome, glandular fever, alcoholism, and drug abuse.

If the immune system is affected, this remedy assists in boosting energy. It was first used with a 56-year-old woman who suffered from full-blown AIDS. She had previously had cancer and was so depleted of vitality she could do nothing for herself. She took Spectrum 12x five times daily for several weeks. After the first week, she reported that she was able to do her housework, wash her hair, and dress herself for the first time in nearly a year. It was at that point that the remedy was given to anyone with serious energy depletion problems.

Roger Savage has potentized it into the higher potencies, and it has as powerful an effect at the higher strengths as it does repeated in low potency. It seems to give stamina and energy at the higher potencies without creating any nervous irritability.

It is suggested that it not be given at night so as not to disturb sleep. It can be given over a long period of time without aggravation, and it seems to have a restorative effect when used for times of stress and exhaustion.

It can be used as a travel remedy as well and gives energy whenever it is used. It helps eliminate the effects of drugs from the aura and, after taking it, people who have had repeated doses of allopathic medicine respond with increased levels of vitality and awareness.

Any substance abuse, which can deplete the body of vitality, will also reflect in the aura as ash or gray. Spectrum vitalizes the entire energetic system and brings color back into the aura. It would be useful for any drug rehabilitation.

Spectrum can be used for:
Physical Problems
It has been used to boost energy in many different diseases. It has helped in pregnancy, labor, and post-partum care. Any degenerative disease responds to it. People with immuno-suppressive diseases have more vitality with its use. Anyone with long-term chronic diseases, where severe pathology exists, would feel better while on the remedy.

Contraindications: None.

Emotional Issues
In people with nervous exhaustion and emotional upset, this remedy gives relief. It helps people handle change and trauma in their lives.

Contraindications: None.

Mental Issues
It revives tired minds and is excellent to take after working with large groups of people or in other situations where energy can be drained.

Contraindications: None.

Essence
The essence of Spectrum is that it provides the energy of all the colors to a worn-out fatigued system. It contains all vibrations within the visible spectrum and provides light to the spirit as well as to the body.

Homeopathic Potency Choices

The color remedies have been potentized by hand at Helios Pharmacy in the following potencies: 3x, 6x, 12x, 18c, 24c, 30c. Roger Savage had taken them up to 200c, 1M, and 10M on his Ray-Potentizer machine. He had success with the higher potencies and has found them particularly useful for acute problems.

All provings were carried out using 30c potencies. The results were varied as to the duration of a remedy. Some symptoms disappeared and never returned, such as gallbladder colic, pains of rheumatoid arthritis, and chronic rhinitis. This is interesting and suggests that the provers were given a dose to match their own constitutional remedy. In other words, it was the vibration and frequency that they needed for their symptoms as much as the similimum remedy that was required. This is the remedy that would be given following the principle of like cures like.

The lower potencies, 3x, and 6x, repeated up to five times a day, have been very useful for all the immunodeficiency cases which were treated with color. The significant mental and emotional symptoms were treated with a single dose of 30c. These were seldom repeated. If there was a need to repeat a color, it was often the color directly higher than the one given rather than a higher potency. For instance, someone whose symptoms disappeared with Yellow would need lime green or a darker green for symptoms that arose subsequently.

Several years ago in India, when the remedies were in their infancy, a single dose of Violet 4x relieved all the symptoms of pain and discomfort an elderly guru had suffered for several years. He felt so good that a second dose of Indigo was given shortly after with the intention of dealing with other symptoms. However, all his original pains returned and he received little benefit when the original Violet was increased to a 6x potency.

That was a useful learning experience and taught me not to change the remedy when a patient is doing well. It showed me how people can react to different vibrations of color remedies.

We can perform muscle-testing or dowse for remedies to find the right potency and how often to repeat it. However, the physical and emotional symptoms can be a better diagnostic tool.

It is hoped that after working with these remedies for awhile, practitioners will be able to supply more information on refining our ability to assess which potencies work best for certain conditions.

It is felt strongly that each potency of a color carries its own particular frequency of healing. The rule of thumb is that physical symptoms respond well to low potencies, and as we progress past 12x, we come into the realms of emotional/mental states. However, since we are dealing with frequencies in the form of color, there is a distinct difference between a Red 30c and Turquoise 3x. There is a hierarchy of incremental change that the colors represent.

It is suggested that a careful study of the chakra system be explored and understood so that the problems and issues which relate to each energy center can be treated with the appropriate potency and color. As we refine our understanding of color and how it works in the human economy, we will better be able to grasp the essential qualities of each potency, as well.

Physical Therapeutics

Red   Pains and irritations with joints and ligaments
                 of the feet, ankles, knees, and hips. Rectal and
                 bowel difficulties, childbirth and post-partum
                 care, varicose veins, piles, circulatory prob-
                 lems, autoimmune deficiency diseases.

Orange   Sexual problems for both sexes, menstrual
                 problems, lower backaches, allergies of all
                 kinds, constipation and sluggish bowels,
                 anorexia and eating disorders, low vitality and
                 post-operative recovery, autoimmume defi-
                 ciency diseases.

Yellow   Liver, gallbladder, stomach, and pancreas
                 problems, absorption problems such as ciliacs,
                 osteoporosis, right eye vision loss, decongestion
                 tion for colds and pulmonary problems, a gen-
                 eral detoxifier.

Green   A general diuretic for edematous tissues, espe-
                 cially suited for pulmonary and cardiac edema.

Cardiac regulator and tonic, detoxifier, calmative, and tranquilizer.

Turquoise A catarrhal remedy, good for sore throats, tired speaking voices, stimulant to the thyroid and parathyroid, good for substance abuse cases where patient wants to stop smoking, drinking, or overeating, neck and shoulder pain.

Indigo Good for tuning the senses: eyes, ears, and nose. Acts as a calmative and anti-insomnia remedy. Good for sinus problems, fevers, congestion to head, such as migraine, and head or eye strain. An anti-inflammatory.

Violet An antiseptic, good for helping wounds heal quickly, a nervous tonic to soothe frayed nerves, improves left eye vision, anti-nausea remedy, acts as a complement in jaundice and liver conditions.

Pink A good remedy for heart patients to ease fears and tension of heart disease; good for new mothers to help increase milk production and attune them to motherhood, a good anti-stress remedy.

Magenta A sexual, heart, and mind remedy which acts as a tonic when energy is low.

Spectrum A general tonic for burn-out, post-viral, or trauma conditions, to be used for substance abuse, overwork, emotional difficulties which drain vitality.

Emotional and Mental Therapeutics

Red   Wherever there is disharmony in vital energy because of feelings of separation due to feeling disconnected from a place, family, or community, when links are weakened, for suicidal and chronic depression, acute and prolonged grief, uprooting.

Orange   Sensual and sexuality difficulties, poverty consciousness, depression, mobility difficulties, very low energy due to depressed states.

Yellow   Ego booster and confidence builder, fearful, agitated, or angry states, increased intelligence, independence, and inner strength.

Green   Peaceful nature and passive spirit, seeking neutrality, avoidance of change, loving and gentle spirits that sometimes become weakened by life.

Turquoise Creative expression, lack of will power to complete tasks, integrity issues, malicious gossipers, liars, timid and shy communicators, those who need to speak up for themselves and express their feelings.

Indigo   Wisdom, discernment, detachment, emotional distance, sensory acuity, imagination, intuition, clarity of thought, tired minds.

Violet   Peace, serenity, beauty, spiritual, ungrounded, weakened ego development, not spiritual, too egotistical, chronic pain dulling perception of life, prejudice.

Pink   Sweetness, softness, want of maternal instincts, tenderness, gentleness, mother love/hate relationships, mothers who can't bond or let go of their children, children who have been neglected or abandoned.

Magenta   High-level thinking and creativity, original, insightful, ready for change, spice of life remedy.

Spectrum   Burn-out on all levels, exhaustion, tension, chronic illness, mental funk.

Afterword

Nearly all the work done on these remedies was done without grants or financial support. Those who offered their time and support did so voluntarily because of their interest in disseminating information to the lay and homeopathic community about the healing properties of color and light.

To investigate these remedies more thoroughly, they need to be used by fellow homeopaths and vibrational and color healers, and their findings thoroughly reported and collated. There is no doubt that these remedies have a capacity to heal. The work on them now needs to be done at more advanced levels not only by homeopaths but also by those interested in the healing power of light as medicine. Anyone interested in understanding the subtle energy system to which these colors relate can enhance their knowledge by studying the chakras and how color works on the human energy system.

If anyone cares to provide information or help of any kind, please have them contact the author. Your support, or useful information would be greatly appreciated.

This book is really an introduction to how potentized light and color can heal. It is an exciting and marvelous exploration that may take a lifetime to complete. If you care to participate in additional provings or wish to purchase a ten-remedy kit of color, please send the request form at the end of this book.

Thank you for reading this book. It is sincerely hoped that you will derive knowledge and benefit from delving into the fascinating world of color. Even at a greatly diluted level, color has tremendous healing power to work for our highest good and greater development. Color is life. It was once said by a wise teacher that we come from color and to color we shall return. It also seems appropriate to say that, while we are in that interim stage called life, we live a colorful and joyful existence.

If you are interested in purchasing a set of the homeopathic color remedies, please send the following to the address below.

1. Your name and address.
2. Specify which potency you wish.
   Sets only come in 6x, 12x, 18c, and 30c.
3. Please include a check or money order for $50 plus $3.00 for postage and handling.

Mail to:
Ambika Wauters, R. S. Hom.
P. O. Box 1371
Boulder, Colorado 80306-1371

If you wish information about the on-line course on Spiritual Homeopathy, workshops, Holistic Healing Holidays, and other products, please contact Ambika at her website at www.ambikawauters.com.

Index

effects of, 13, 14, 15
potentized, 17
"like curing like" principle,
15, 33

M
Magenta, 25, 43, 57, 72, 76,
78, 111, 115-117, 124,
125
used for emotional issues,
117
used for essences, 117
used for homeopathic
related remedies, 117
used for mental issues,
117
used for physical prob-
lems, 116
meditation, 38, 72
mental therapeutics, 125-
126
Morgan, John, 24

N
Nadis, 45
Native Americans, 68, 69,
82, 100
Newton, Sir Isaac, 31

O
Orange, 25, 27, 41, 43, 46,
49, 55, 63, 77, 81-88, 113,
114, 123, 125
used for emotional issues,
87
used for essences, 88
used for homeopathic
related remedies, 88
used for mental issues, 87
used for physical prob-
lems, 86

P
physical therapeutics, 123-
124
Pink, 20, 22, 41, 42, 43, 47,
63, 64, 67, 85, 97, 112-
114, 124, 125
used for emotional issues,
114
used for essences, 114
used for homeopathic
related remedies, 114
used for mental issues,
114
used for physical prob-
lems, 113
Principles of Color Healing,
The, 114

V

vibrational healing, 15, 17, 36

vibrational medicine, 34

Violet, 16, 25, 43, 72, 76, 78, 93, 107-112, 121, 124, 125
  used for emotional issues, 111
  used for essences, 112
  used for mental issues, 111
  used for physical problems, 110

W

Watson, Ian, 18, 19

Winter Solstice, 18, 19, 24, 25

Y

Yeats, William Butler, 74

Yellow, 25, 28, 46, 65, 88-94, 121, 123, 125
  used for emotional issues, 93
  used for essences, 94
  used for homeopathic related remedies, 94
  used for mental issues, 93
  used for physical problems, 92

BOOKS BY THE CROSSING PRESS

Chakras and Their Archetypes: *Uniting Energy Awareness and Spiritual Growth*
By Ambika Wauters

Linking classic archetypes to the seven chakras in the human energy system can reveal unconscious ways of behaving. Wauters helps us understand where our energy is blocked, which attitudes or emotional issues are responsible, and how to then transcend our limitations.

$16.95 • Paper • ISBN 0-89594-891-5

Healing with the Energy of the Chakras
By Ambika Wauters

Chakras are swirling wheels of light and color—vortices through which energy must pass in order to nourish and maintain physical, emotional, mental and spiritual life. Wauters presents a self-help program intended to give you guidelines and a framework within which to explore and understand more about how your energetic system responds to thoughts and expression.

$14.95 • Paper • ISBN 0-89594-906-7

Color and Crystals: *A Journey Through the Chakras*
By Joy Gardner-Gordon

Information about color, crystals, tones, personality types, and Tarot archetypes that correspond to each chakra. Fully illustrated, indexed and well-organized.

$14.95 • Paper • ISBN 0-89594-258-5

BOOKS BY THE CROSSING PRESS

Essential Reiki: *A Complete Guide to an Ancient Healing Art*

By Diane Stein

This bestseller includes the history of Reiki, hand positions, giving treatments, and the initiations. While no book can replace directly received attunements, Essential Reiki provides everything else that the practitioner and teacher of this system needs, including all three degrees of Reiki, most of it in print for the first time.

$18.95 • Paper • ISBN 0-89594-736-6

Healing with Color Zone Therapy

By Joseph Corvo and Lilian Verner-Bonds

Corvo and Verner-Bonds introduce a form of therapy that treats the whole person: the physical, the emotional, and the spiritual. The safe, step-by-step techniques of Color Zone Therapy are followed by an A-Z list of charts for more than one hundred common ailments.

$14.95 • Paper • ISBN 0-89594-925-3

The Healing Energy of Your Hands

By Michael Bradford

Bradford offers techniques so simple that anyone can work with healing energy quickly and easily.

$12.95 • Paper • ISBN 0-89594-781-1

BOOKS BY THE CROSSING PRESS

The Sevenfold Journey: *Reclaiming Mind, Body & Spirit Through the Chakras*
By Anodea Judith & Selene Vega

Combining yoga, movement, psychotherapy, and ritual, the authors weave ancient and modern wisdom into a powerful tapestry of techniques for facilitating personal growth and healing.

$18.95 • Paper • ISBN 0-89594-574-6

Your Body Speaks Your Mind: *How Your thoughts and Emotions Affect Your Health*
By Debbie Shapiro

Debbie Shapiro examines the intimate connection between the mind and body revealing insights into how our unresolved thoughts and feelings affect our health and manifest as illness in specific parts of the body.

$14.95 • Paper • ISBN 0-89594-893-1

To receive a current catalog from The Crossing Press
please call toll-free, 800-777-1048.
www. crossingpress.com